Pet Owner Educational Atlas

DIGESTIVE SYSTEM

Texts and review: Sarah M. Schmid • M. Katherine Tolbert

edra
PUBLISHING

Pet Owner Educational Atlas. Digestive System
Sarah M. Schmid and M. Katherine Tolbert

ISBN: 978-1-957260-28-0
eISBN: 978-1-957260-48-8

Illustrator: Jacob Gragera Artal, Grupo Asís Biomedia S.L., Zaragoza, Spain
Cover, Layout and Copyediting: Grupo Asís Biomedia S.L., Zaragoza, Spain
Project Manager: Jorge Viejo Adiego, Grupo Asís Biomedia S.L., Zaragoza, Spain

Edra Publishing US LLC
3309 Northlake Boulevard, Suite 203
Palm Beach Gardens, FL, 33403
EIN: 844113980
info@edrapublishing.com
www.edrapublishing.com

edra
PUBLISHING

Printed by *"Imprenta Mundo" S.L.U., Cambre (A Coruña)*, Spain, October 2022

PREFACE

Gastrointestinal signs such as vomiting, diarrhea, changes in appetite, and weight loss are a common complaint in dogs and cats presenting to a veterinarian. Although these clinical signs are not specific to any one disease, they are often associated with ailments of the gastrointestinal tract, liver, gallbladder, or pancreas. Together, these organs make up the digestive system.

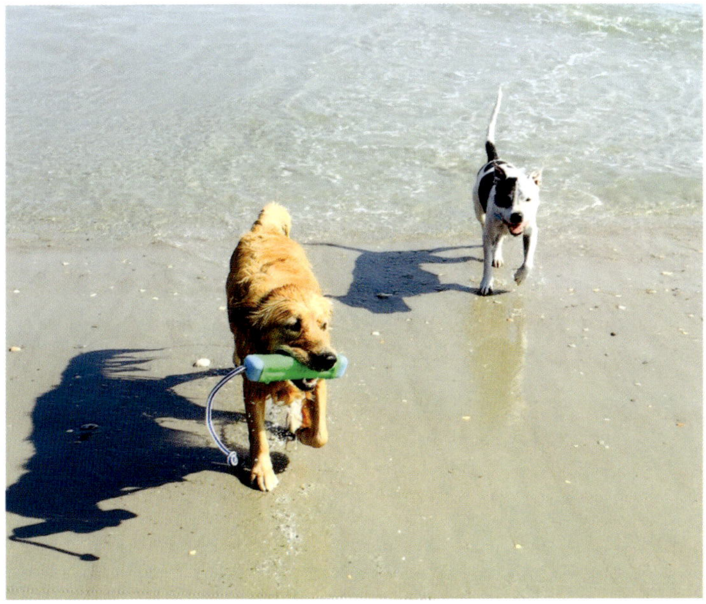

Dante*, and his best friend* Lady Bird*, in his favorite environment*

Through the use of detailed illustrations and concise explanations, this atlas has been designed as a comprehensive tool to facilitate communication between the veterinarian and the pet owner. The collaboration of the owner is essential during both the diagnosis and treatment of disease. This is especially true for diseases such as chronic enteropathy in which strict therapeutic trials are needed to achieve a diagnosis, as a single test is unlikely to yield a definitive diagnosis.

It is important to recognize that the diagnostic and therapeutic approach to gastrointestinal disorders relies on proper localization of the disease, which can often be discerned from the history. For example, the diagnostic approach to a dog with regurgitation is quite different to that of a dog that is vomiting. However, to the untrained eye of a pet owner, regurgitation may be difficult to distinguish from vomiting. Similarly, the diagnostic approaches to large bowel diarrhea and small bowel diarrhea are different. To facilitate gathering these key points of information, the book includes a section outlining the diagnostic approach to gastrointestinal diseases.

The content of this atlas is organized into three major organ systems: the gastrointestinal tract, the hepatobiliary system, and the pancreas. Each of these sections begins with an overview of normal anatomy and physiology, highlighting key anatomical features and functions. This is followed by a summary of the most common diseases affecting each organ system, including the most relevant information about clinical signs, diagnosis, treatment, and prognosis. Finally, various procedures of the gastrointestinal and hepatobiliary systems are described.

This atlas is the result of the work of an extraordinary team coordinated by Jorge Viejo, with vivid illustrations by Jacob Gragera. This team has been so supportive in helping us design our vision with great skill and elegance. We are happy we **trusted our gut** and joined the team at Grupo Asís to create a truly unique resource for digestive diseases of the dog and cat. Finally, we would like to dedicate our work on this atlas to *Dante*, a loyal Pit Bull mix whose gastric cancer took him far too soon.

We hope that you find this atlas a valuable tool to facilitate your learning, teach your team, and communicate with pet owners.

Sarah M. Schmid, DVM, DACVIM (SAIM)
Assistant professor, University of Tennessee, USA

M. Katherine Tolbert, DVM, PhD, DACVIM (SAIM)
Clinical associate professor, Texas A&M University, USA

Table of contents

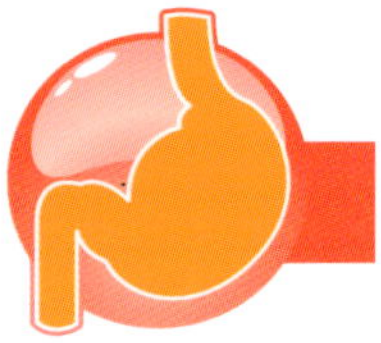

01 ANATOMY AND PHYSIOLOGY OF THE GASTROINTESTINAL TRACT

1 Anatomy of the gastrointestinal tract 7
2 Gastric mucosal barrier 8
3 Gastrointestinal nervous system 9
4 Gastrointestinal endocrinology 10

02 DIAGNOSTIC APPROACH TO GASTROINTESTINAL DISEASES

5 Regurgitation vs. vomiting 11
6 Small vs. large bowel diarrhea 12
7 Weight loss in the face of polyphagia 13

03 DISEASES OF THE GASTROINTESTINAL TRACT

Diseases of the esophagus

8 Esophagitis 14
9 Esophageal stricture 15
10 Vascular ring anomalies 16
11 Megaesophagus (ME) 17
12 Hiatal hernia 18
13 Gastroesophageal reflux 19

Diseases of the stomach

14 Acute gastritis 20
15 Chronic gastritis 21
16 Gastric dilatation and volvulus (GDV) 22
17 Delayed gastric emptying 23
18 Gastroduodenal ulcers 24

Diseases of the small intestine

19 Acute enteritis 25
20 Acute hemorrhagic diarrheal syndrome (AHDS) 26
21 Canine parvovirus infection 27
22 Intestinal dysbiosis 28
23 Chronic enteropathy 29
24 Intestinal lymphangiectasia 30
25 Feline inflammatory bowel disease vs. small-cell lymphoma 31

Diseases of the large intestine

26 Acute colitis 32
27 Infectious colitis 33
28 Idiopathic chronic colitis 34
29 Granulomatous colitis 35
30 Feline constipation and megacolon 36

Diseases of the rectum and anus

31 Anal sac impaction and infection 37
32 Perianal fistula 38
33 Apocrine gland anal sac adenocarcinoma (AGASACA) 39

Miscellaneous gastrointestinal diseases

34 Gastrointestinal foreign bodies 40
35 Intussusception 41
36 Gastrointestinal parasites 42
37 Gastrointestinal cancer 43
38 Acute abdomen 44

04 GASTROINTESTINAL PROCEDURES

39 Upper gastrointestinal endoscopy 45
40 Ileal intubation and biopsy 46
41 Colonoscopy 47
42 Feeding tubes 48
43 Esophageal balloon dilatation 49
44 Fecal microbiota transplantation (FMT) 50

05 ANATOMY AND PHYSIOLOGY OF THE HEPATOBILIARY SYSTEM

45 Anatomy of the hepatobiliary system 51
46 Regulation of bile secretion 52

06 DISEASES OF THE HEPATOBILIARY SYSTEM

Diseases of the gallbladder and bile ducts

47 Cholecystitis 53
48 Gallbladder mucocele 54
49 Cholelithiasis and choledocholithiasis 55
50 Extrahepatic bile duct obstruction (EHBDO) 56
51 Biliary cancer 57

Diseases of the liver

52 Congenital portosystemic shunt (cPSS) 58
53 Hepatic arteriovenous malformation (HAVM) 59
54 Canine acute hepatitis 60
55 Vacuolar hepatopathy 61
56 Canine chronic hepatitis 62
57 Copper-associated hepatopathy 63
58 Cirrhosis 64
59 Hepatocutaneous syndrome 65
60 Feline neutrophilic cholangitis 66
61 Feline lymphocytic cholangitis 67
62 Feline triaditis 68
63 Feline hepatic lipidosis 69
64 Hepatic cancer 70

07 HEPATOBILIARY PROCEDURES

65 Cholecystocentesis 71
66 Laparoscopic liver biopsy 72

08 ANATOMY AND PHYSIOLOGY OF THE PANCREAS

67 Anatomy of the pancreas 73
68 Physiology of the pancreas 74

09 DISEASES OF THE PANCREAS

69 Exocrine pancreatic insufficiency (EPI) 75
70 Acute pancreatitis 76
71 Chronic pancreatitis 77
72 Pancreatic abscesses and pseudocysts 78
73 Pancreatic cancer 79

1 Anatomy of the gastrointestinal tract

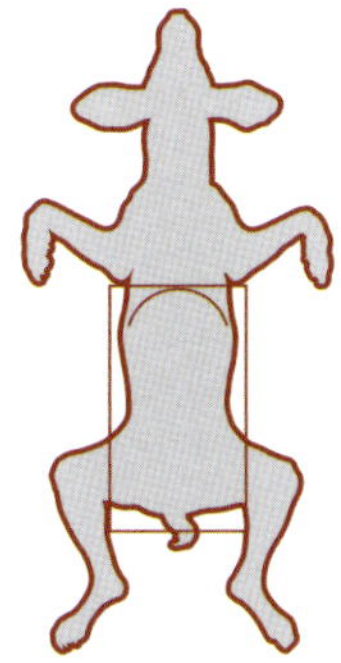

1. Liver
2. Stomach
3. Spleen
4. Greater omentum
5. Esophagus
6. Diaphragm
7. Pylorus
8. Descending duodenum
9. Jejunum
10. Ileum
11. Cecum
12. Ascending colon
13. Transverse colon
14. Descending colon
15. Urinary bladder
16. Pancreas
17. Gallbladder
18. Major duodenal papilla
19. Minor duodenal papilla

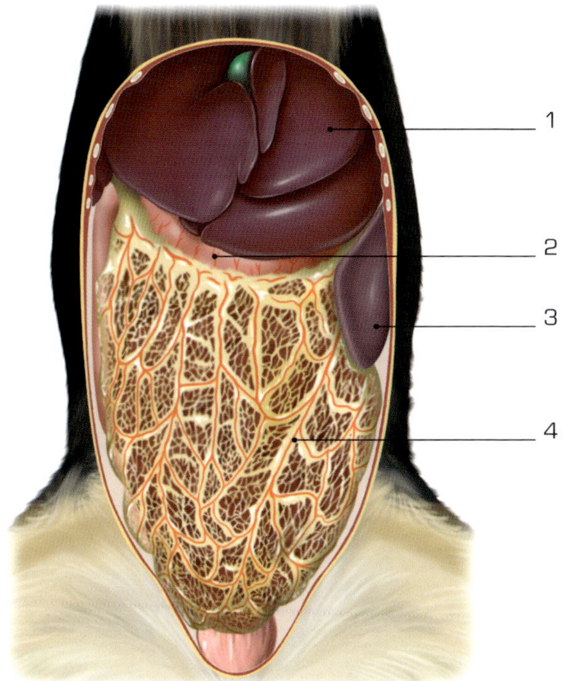

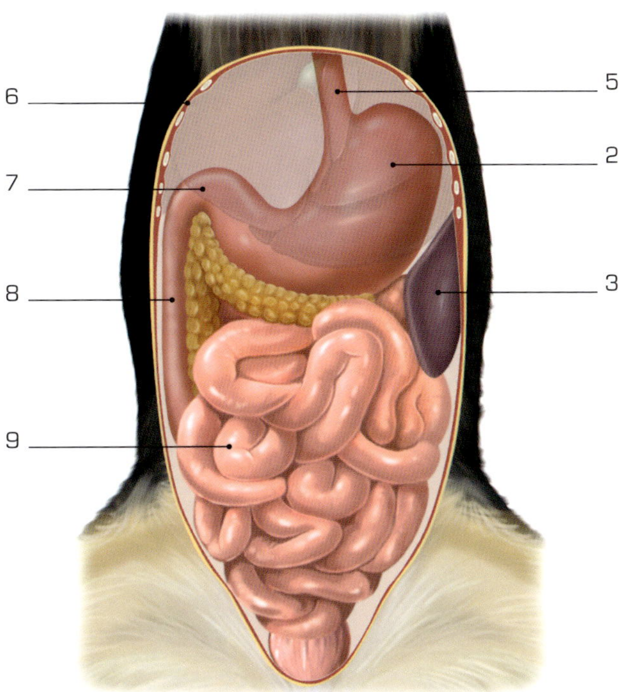

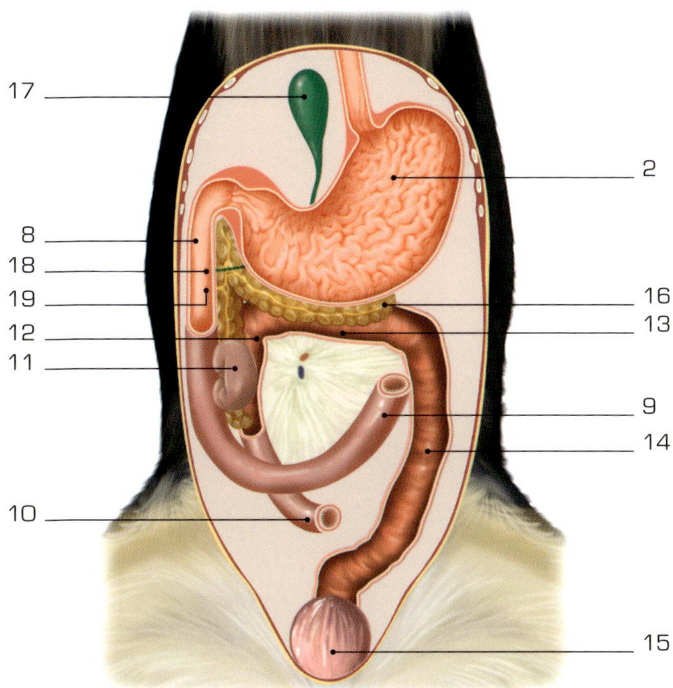

2 Gastric mucosal barrier

The gastric mucosal barrier keeps hydrochloric acid and digestive enzymes contained within the lumen of the stomach.

Mucus–bicarbonate barrier

- 5–200 μm thick layer composed of mucopolysaccharides, glycoproteins, and water.
- Secreted by mucous neck cells in parietal glands and gastric epithelial cells.
- Superficial water-soluble mucus acts as a lubricant to prevent mechanical damage.
- Adherent layer is impermeable to large proteins (protection against peptic proteolysis).

Single layer of columnar epithelial cells

- Tight junctions between cells.
- Hydrophobic phospholipids within the apical membrane repel gastric acid.
- Generation of prostaglandins (PGE_2, PGI_2).
- Mucosal bicarbonate secretion ("alkaline tide").

Gastric mucosal blood flow

- Regulation of local acid–base balance.

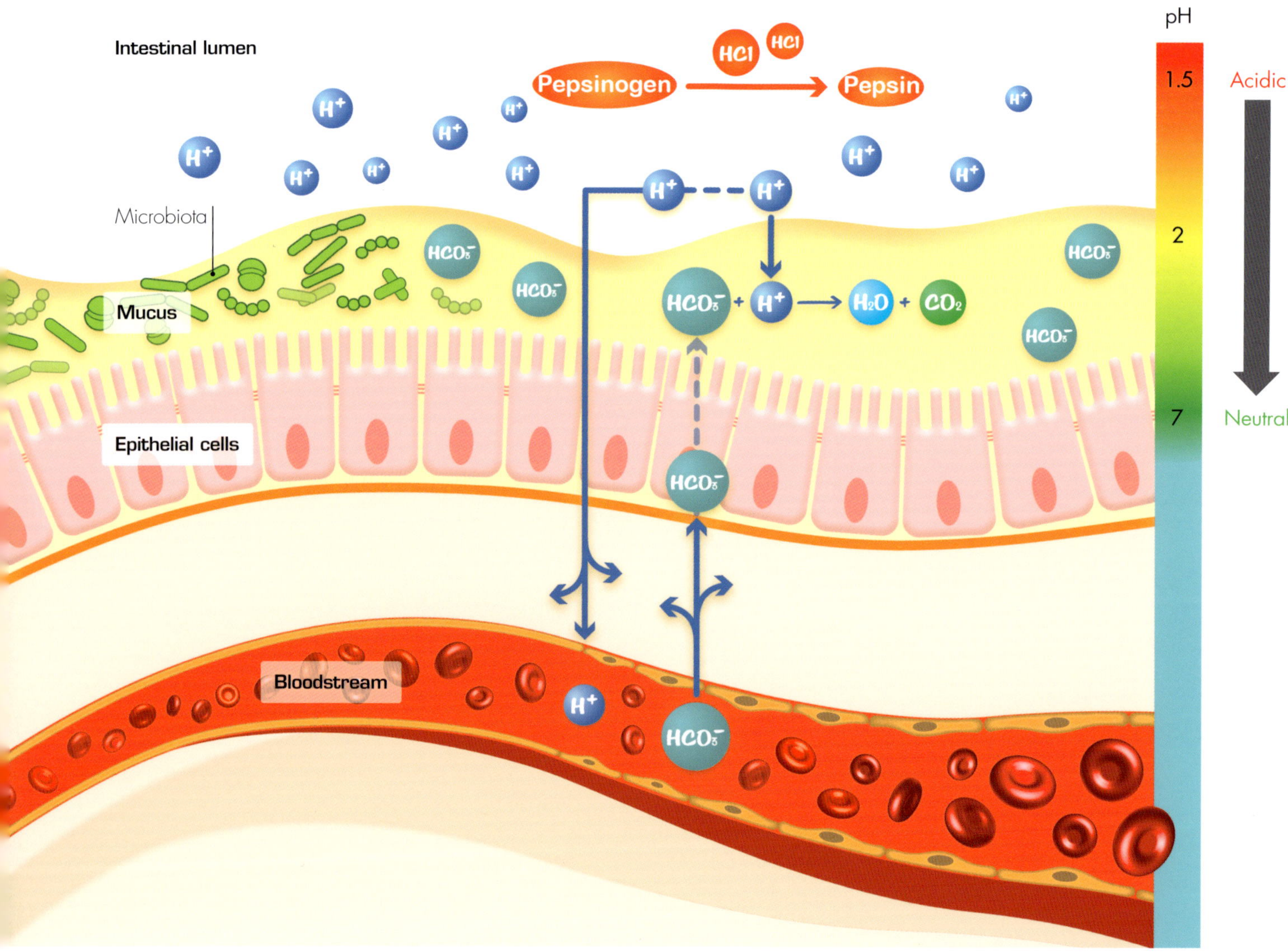

3 Gastrointestinal nervous system

Extrinsic nervous system

The extrinsic nervous system consists of parasympathetic and sympathetic branches. In general, parasympathetic fibers are stimulatory and sympathetic fibers are inhibitory to the gastrointestinal tract. One exception is that sympathetic fibers are excitatory to the muscularis mucosa.

- **Parasympathetic innervation:** acetylcholine from the vagus nerve (upper gastrointestinal tract) and pelvic nerve (lower gastrointestinal tract).
- **Sympathetic innervation:** norepinephrine from the spinal cord (T1–L3 segments).

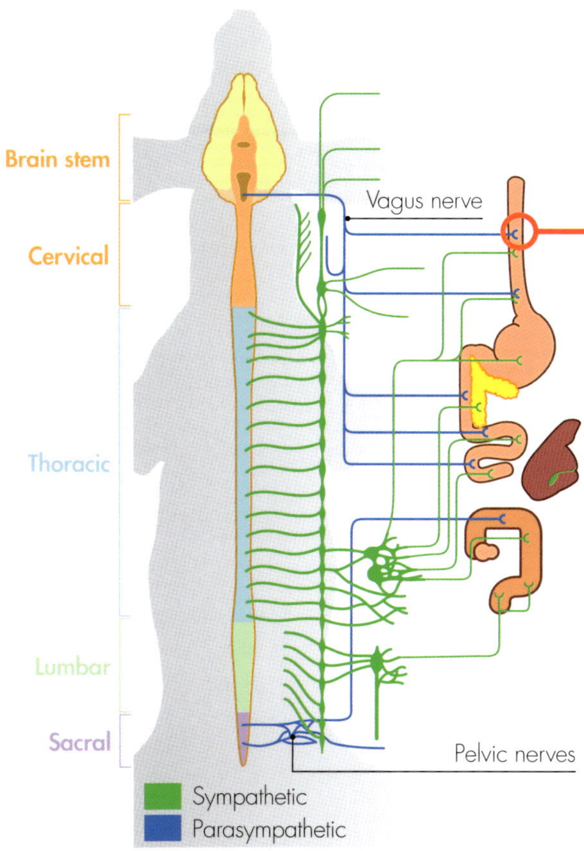

Intrinsic (enteric) nervous system

The intrinsic nervous system has ganglia located in the submucosal and myenteric plexuses.

- **Myenteric plexus:** controls muscle activity and movement along the gastrointestinal tract.
- **Submucosal plexus:** controls local intestinal secretion, absorption, and contraction of submucosal muscle.

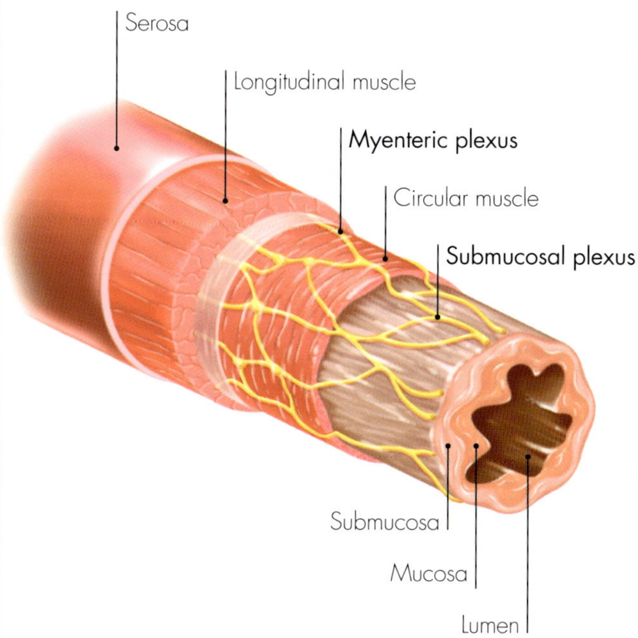

Given that the parasympathetic nervous system is stimulatory to the gastrointestinal tract, pharmacologic intervention for ileus includes parasympathomimetics such as cisapride, bethanechol, and, indirectly, metoclopramide.

4 Gastrointestinal endocrinology

Enteroendocrine cells secrete various hormones that aid in gastric acid production and inhibition, pancreatic secretion, gallbladder contraction, insulin secretion, and gastrointestinal motility.

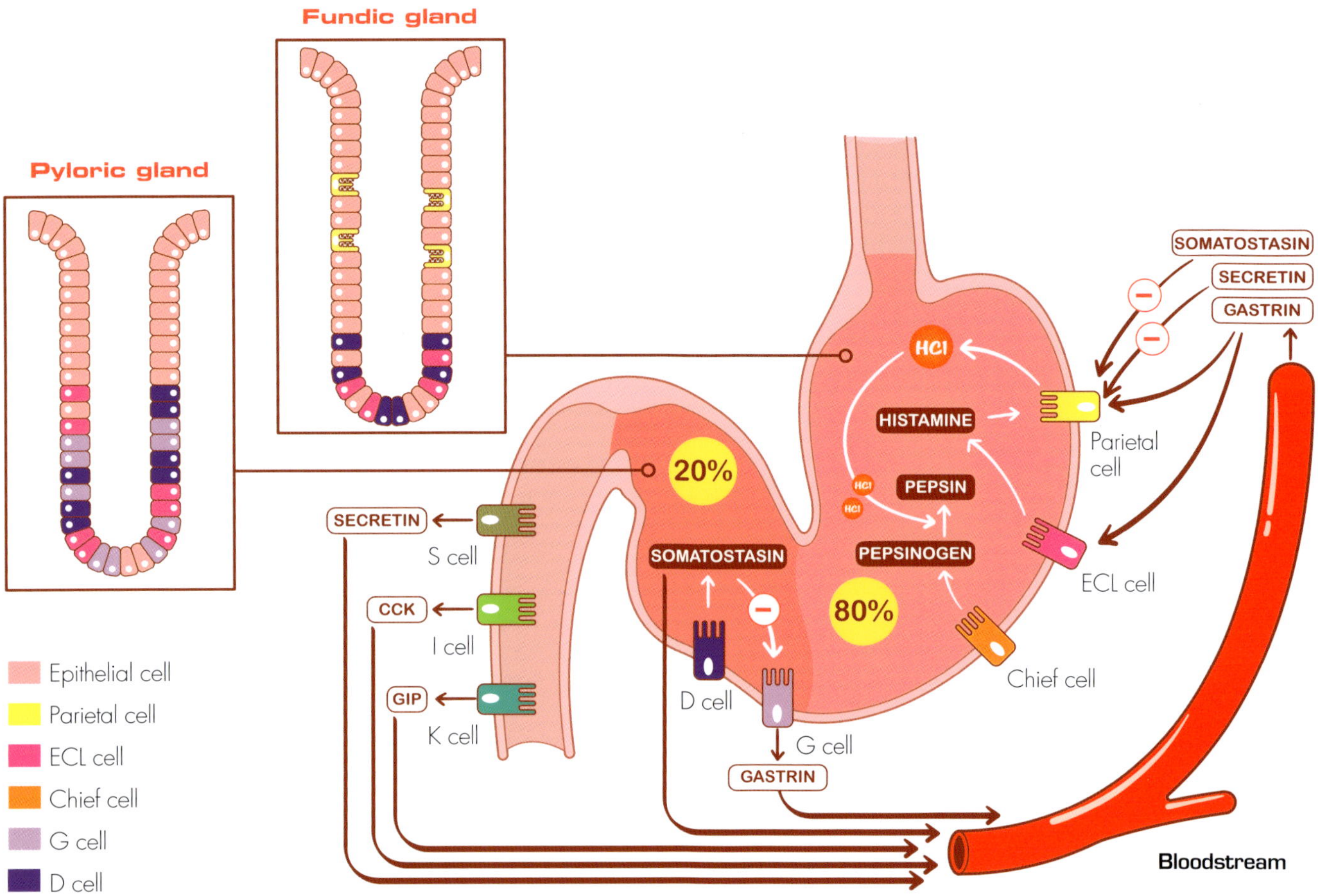

Hormone	Stimulus	Site of action	Action
Gastrin G cells	Intragastric peptides Gastric distension	Parietal cells	H^+ secretion
Histamine ECL cells	Gastrin	Parietal cells	H^+ secretion
Pepsinogen Chief cells	Hydrochloric acid (HCl)	Gastric lumen	Converted to pepsin to begin protein digestion
Somatostatin D cells	H^+ (decreased gastric pH as food moves out of stomach)	G cells Parietal cells	Inhibition of G cells Inhibition of parietal cells Decreased gastric motility
Secretin S cells	Low duodenal pH	Parietal cells Pancreatic ductal cells	Inhibition of acid secretion Secretion of HCO_3^--rich pancreatic fluid Delay of gastric emptying
Cholecystokinin (CCK) I cells	Intraduodenal fatty acids, amino acids, H^+	Pancreas Gallbladder	Pancreatic enzyme secretion Gallbladder contraction

5 Regurgitation vs. vomiting

The diagnostic approach to vomiting and regurgitation varies considerably. Consequently, it is important to differentiate these two processes. In contrast to regurgitation, vomiting involves a centrally mediated reflux with coordinated closure of the nasopharynx and glottis to protect the airway, thereby reducing the risk for aspiration pneumonia. Both vomiting and regurgitation must also be differentiated from expectoration (expulsion of material associated with coughing).

! Ask yourself: would I be able to move out a rug from in front of the dog before expulsion of material? If the answer is yes, it is likely vomiting.

! There is often warning when a dog is about to vomit. Conversely, in case of regurgitation, the dog seems to simply lower its head and material comes out.

Regurgitation

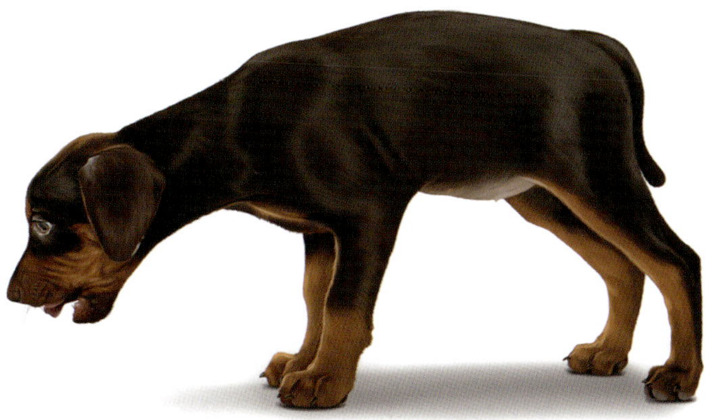

Vomiting

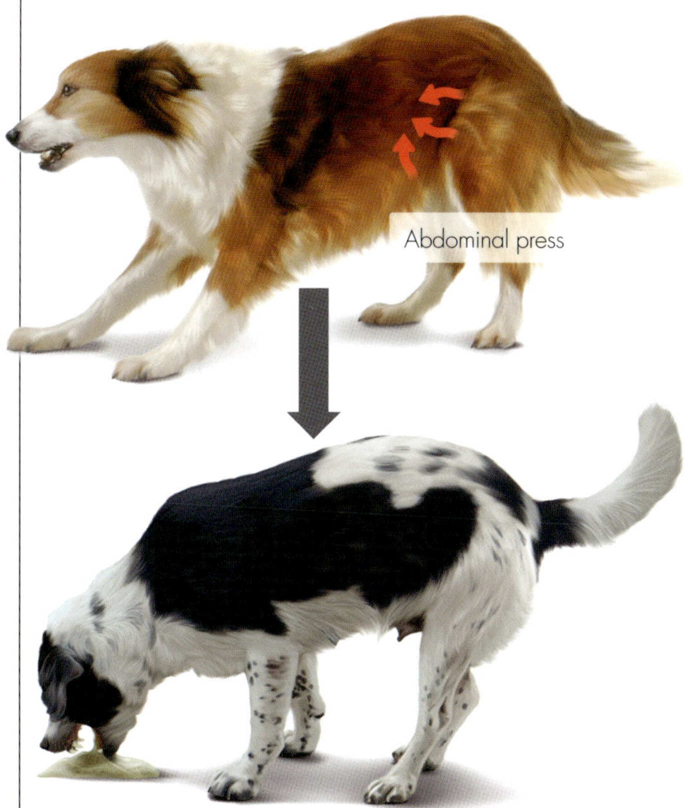

	Regurgitation	Vomiting
Definition	**Passive** expulsion of food, fluid, or other material	**Active** expulsion of ingesta from the stomach (and sometimes the duodenum)
Localization	Esophagus	Caudal to the gastroesophageal sphincter (stomach, small intestines)
Nausea	Absent (except in painful conditions)	Common (lip smacking, salivation)
Retching	Absent	Present (active movement of abdominal muscles)
Bile	Absent	May or may not be present
Volume	Any	Any
Causes	Vascular ring anomaly, stricture, esophageal foreign body, esophageal cancer, esophagitis, megaesophagus, gastroesophageal reflux, gastroesophageal intussusception, hiatal hernia	Systemic, metabolic, or endocrine disease: pancreatitis, liver disease, kidney disease, hyperthyroidism, hypoadrenocorticism Primary gastrointestinal disease: infectious (parasitic, viral, fungal), inflammatory, cancerous, toxic

6 Small vs. large bowel diarrhea

When differentiating small from large bowel diarrhea, it is helpful to think about the function of each part of the gastrointestinal tract. The small intestinal villi and prominent brush border microvilli are important for the digestion and absorption of nutrients and water. Consequently, weight loss, polyphagia, and large-volume diarrhea may result with small intestinal disease. In contrast, the large intestine plays a role in extracting remaining water and electrolytes and controlling defecation. Thus, large bowel diarrhea is characterized by signs of decreased ability to store and control defecation. Although mucus can be seen in both types of diarrhea, the presence of mucus is most often a sign of large bowel diarrhea.

Determining whether diarrhea originates from the small or large intestine is key to assembling a differential list and diagnostic plan.

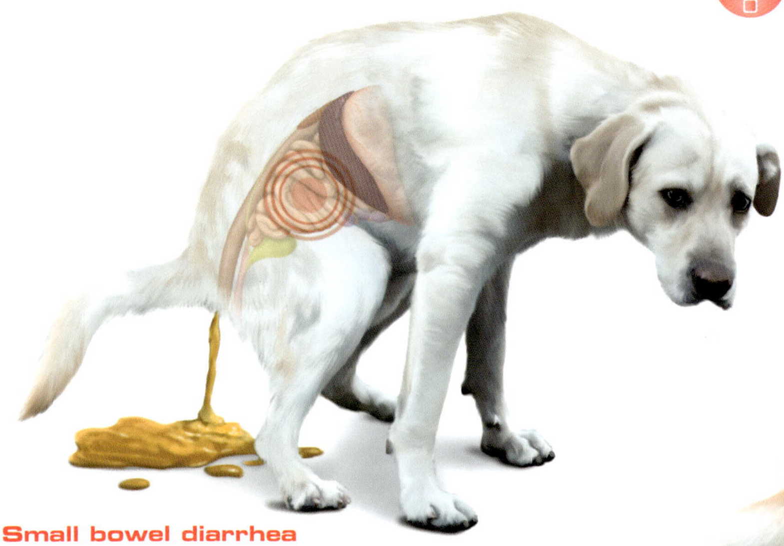

Small bowel diarrhea

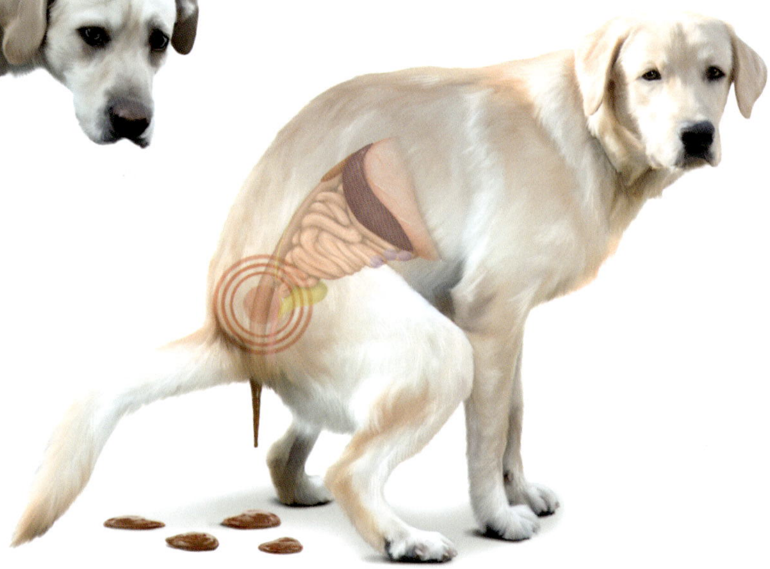

Large bowel diarrhea

	Small bowel diarrhea Digestion and absorption	**Large bowel diarrhea** Storage and continence
Weight loss	May be present	Absent
Polyphagia (increased appetite)	May be present	Absent
Tenesmus (straining to defecate)	Absent	Present
Frequency	Normal	↑ or normal
Volume	↑ or normal	↓ or normal
Blood	Melena (dark, tarry —i.e., digested— blood)	Hematochezia (frank red blood)
Mucus	Small amounts may be present	Present
Vomiting	May be present	Uncommon

7 Weight loss in the face of polyphagia

Weight loss must first be defined in the context of appetite and energy intake. For example, if a pet is eating less (e.g., due to hyporexia), weight loss is expected. However, weight loss despite eating a normal or increased amount (i.e., polyphagia) is inappropriate and indicates either a decrease in caloric intake, maldigestion and/or malabsorption, or an increase in metabolism or catabolism.

> The diagnostic workup for weight loss in the face of a good appetite can be approached by ruling out problems in normal digestion, absorption, and metabolism.

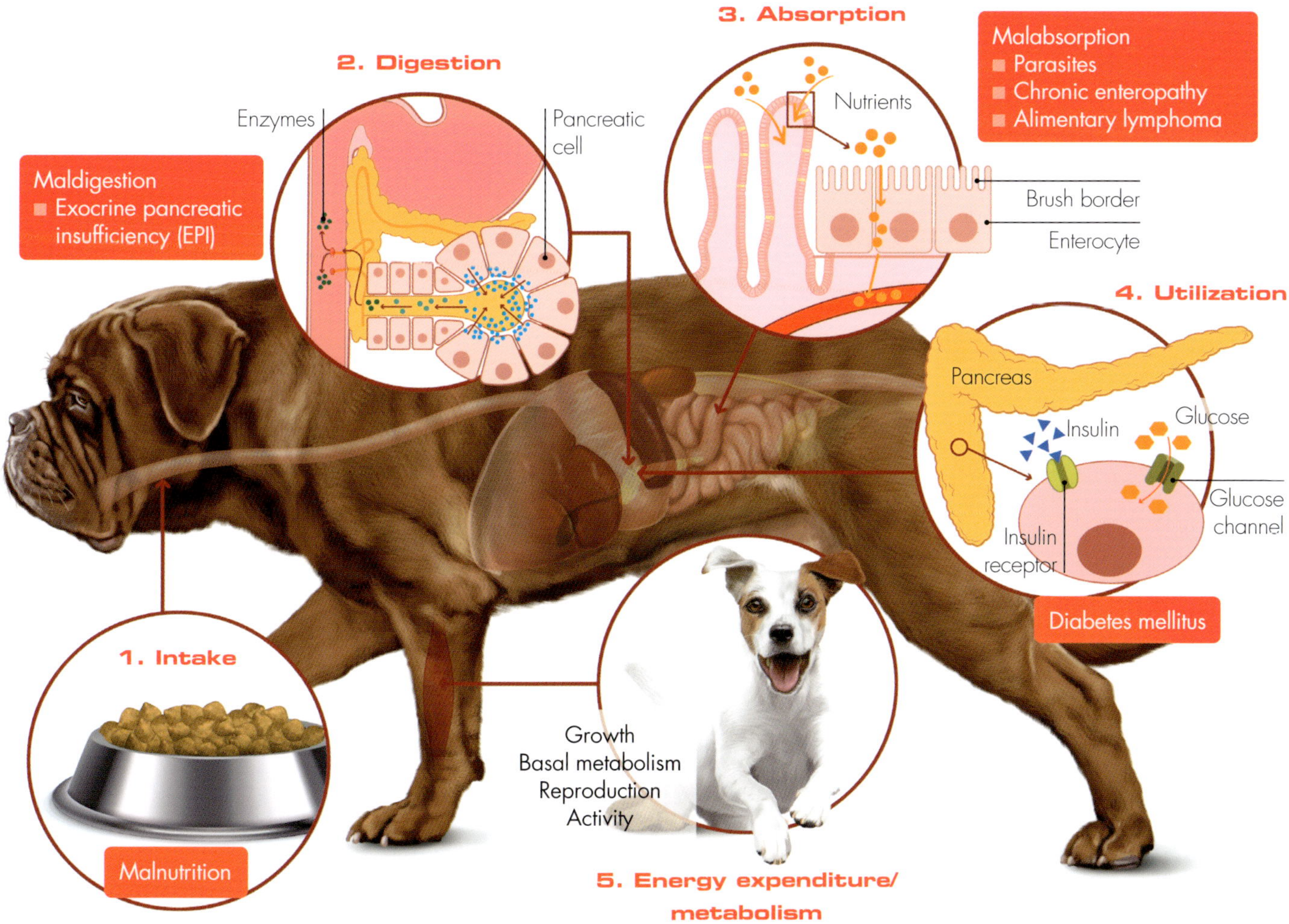

RER = 70 × (weight in kg)$^{0.75}$
DER = life stage factor × RER

Energy-consumptive processes
- Hyperthyroidism (cats)
- Cancer cachexia
- Cardiac cachexia
- Increase in exercise

DER, daily energy requirement
RER, resting energy requirement

DISEASES OF THE ESOPHAGUS

8 Esophagitis

Esophagitis is an acute or chronic inflammatory disorder of the esophageal mucosa (inner lining of the esophagus). It may result from a variety of causes including foreign bodies, severe chronic vomiting, ingestion of caustic agents or drugs (e.g., doxycycline, clindamycin), gastroesophageal reflux during anesthesia, and secondary to a hiatal hernia.

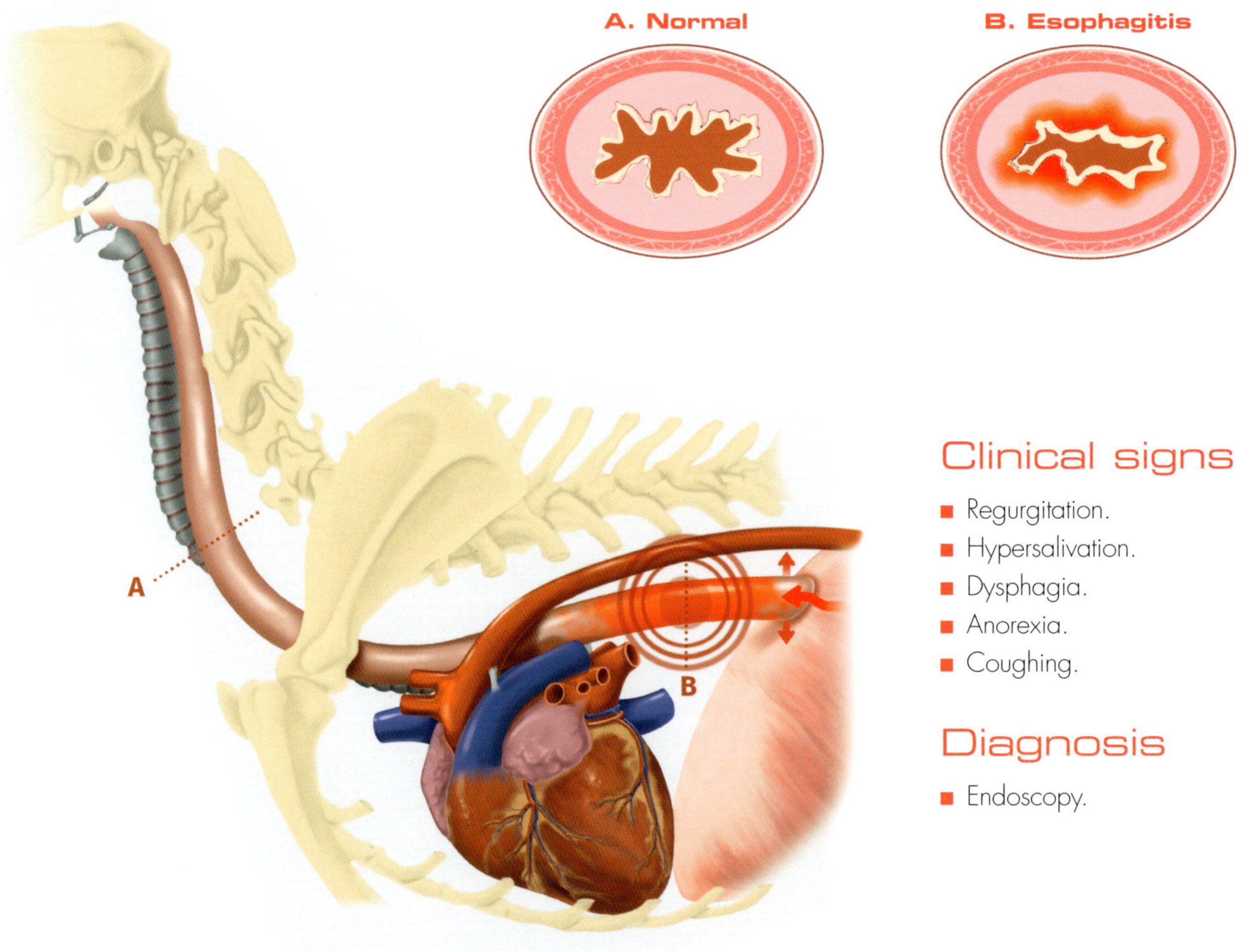

Clinical signs

- Regurgitation.
- Hypersalivation.
- Dysphagia.
- Anorexia.
- Coughing.

Diagnosis

- Endoscopy.

Treatment

- Sucralfate slurry to protect the esophageal mucosa and reduce pain.
- Proton pump inhibitors (omeprazole) to reduce the acidity of gastroesophageal reflux fluids.
- Low-fat, low-fiber, canned food in small frequent meals to decrease gastric content by increasing gastric emptying.
- Systemic analgesics for pain management.
- Cisapride (or metoclopramide) to increase the tone of the lower esophageal sphincter.
- Treatment of underlying causes: foreign bodies, chronic vomiting.

Prognosis

- Time to resolution of clinical signs: from 5–7 days (mild cases) to ≥3 weeks (severe cases).
- Severe esophagitis may lead to esophageal stricture formation.

DISEASES OF THE ESOPHAGUS

9 Esophageal stricture

An esophageal stricture is an abnormal narrowing of the esophageal lumen. The narrowing can be so severe that food may not be able to pass. As a potential complication of severe esophagitis, stricture formation can result from ingestion of caustic substances and trauma from esophageal foreign bodies. However, some strictures may form secondary to intraluminal or extraluminal masses (e.g., cancer, abscesses). *Spirocerca lupi* infections have been associated with the development of esophageal sarcomas.

Clinical signs

- Regurgitation.
- Hypersalivation.
- Dysphagia, odynophagia.
- Coughing.
- Weight loss despite polyphagia.

Diagnosis

- Barium esophagram.
- Videofluoroscopic swallow studies.
- Endoscopy.

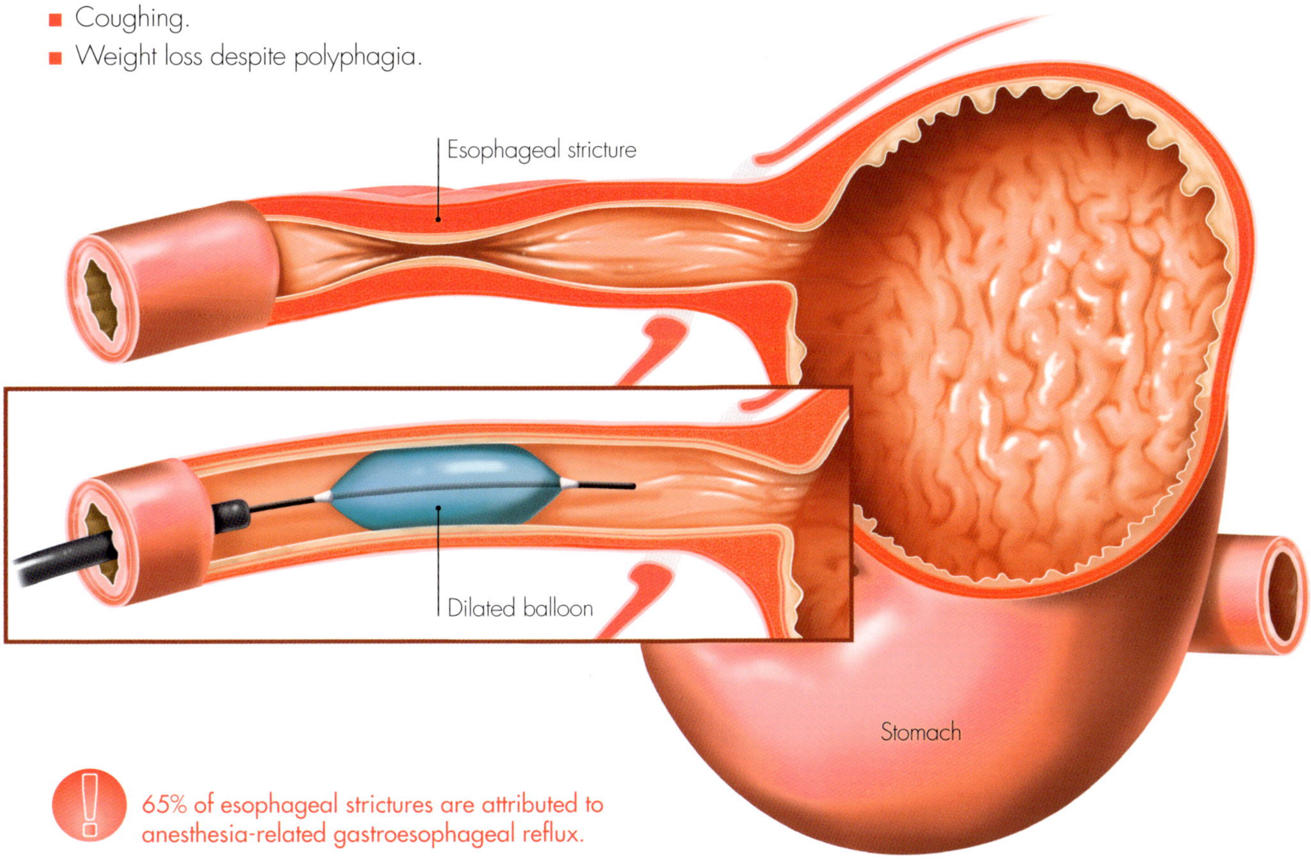

65% of esophageal strictures are attributed to anesthesia-related gastroesophageal reflux.

Treatment

- Endoscopically ± fluoroscopically guided balloon dilatation or bougienage. Multiple procedures are generally required. Transendoscopic triamcinolone injections and/or oral steroid therapy after dilatation.
- An indwelling balloon dilatation esophagostomy tube may be considered.
- Refractory strictures may require placement of a gastrostomy feeding tube; however, this does not prevent regurgitation of swallowed salivary secretions, which can result in aspiration pneumonia.
- Treatment of esophagitis (see Sheet 8).

Prognosis

- 70%–80% of patients respond to balloon dilatation.
- Life-threatening esophageal perforation may occur when attempting dilatation.

DISEASES OF THE ESOPHAGUS

10 Vascular ring anomalies

Vascular ring anomalies are congenital (birth) malformations of the major arteries of the heart that result in an entrapped esophagus, causing obstruction. Most puppies and kittens present as they transition to solid foods. The most common type of vascular ring anomaly in the dog is a persistent right aortic arch (PRAA), which occurs when the embryonic right aortic arch becomes the functional aorta rather than the left fourth aortic arch. As a result, the esophagus becomes trapped between the right-sided aorta, the pulmonary artery, and the ligamentum arteriosum.

Clinical signs

- Regurgitation at the time of weaning.
- Weight loss despite a good appetite.
- Failure to thrive.
- Signs of aspiration pneumonia (coughing, dyspnea, fever).

Diagnosis

- Thoracic radiographs reveal esophageal dilatation just before the base of the heart (often seen with a barium swallow study).
- CT scan.

Careful cardiac auscultation is key, as many dogs with a PRAA may have a heart murmur secondary to a concurrent patent ductus arteriosus (PDA).

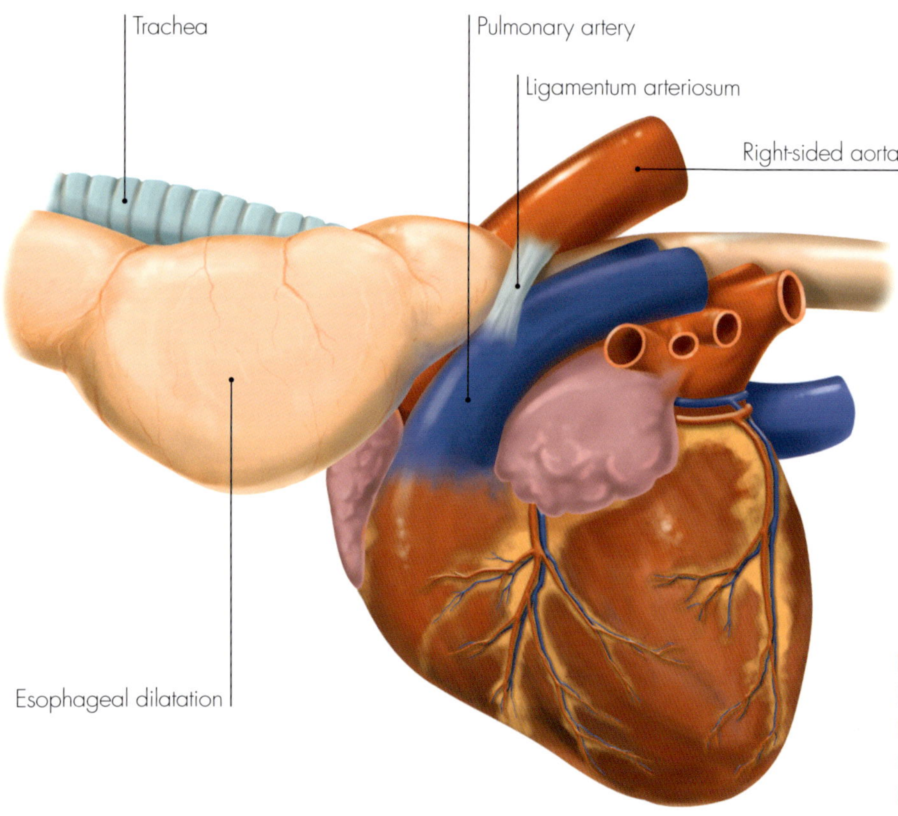

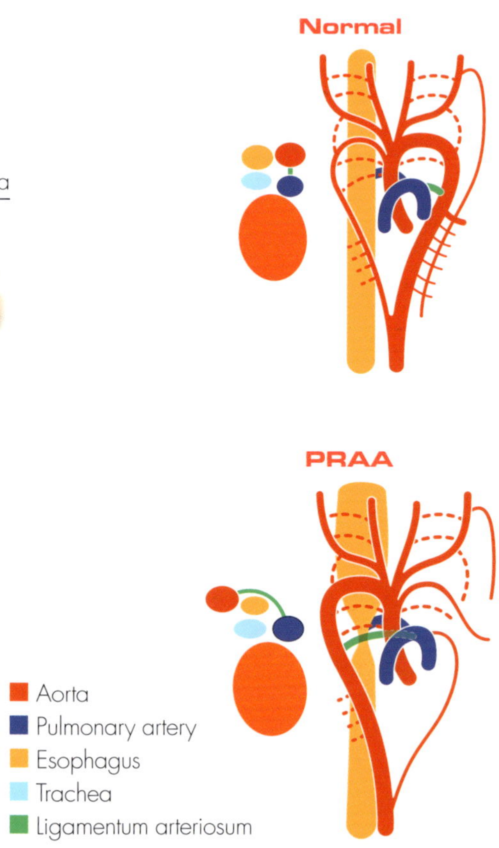

Treatment

- Surgery: transection of the ligamentum arteriosum.
- Malnourished animals may require nutritional support via gastrostomy tubes prior to surgery.
- Upright feeding of various consistencies of food is indicated prior to surgery (see Sheet 11).

Prognosis

- Clinical improvement in 90% of patients following surgery.
- Fibrosis and strictures may occur prior to surgery.
- Esophageal hypomotility and regurgitation may persist.

DISEASES OF THE ESOPHAGUS

11 Megaesophagus (ME)

ME is a disorder in which the esophagus dilates and loses motility. When motility is decreased or absent, food and liquid have difficulty being propelled into the stomach and accumulate within the esophagus. ME can be congenital (at birth) or acquired secondary to myasthenia gravis, hypoadrenocorticism (Addison's disease), polymyopathies, polyneuropathies, dysautonomia, lead poisoning, or severe esophagitis. Idiopathic acquired ME is most common.

Clinical signs

- Regurgitation.
- Malnutrition.
- Signs of aspiration pneumonia (coughing, difficulty breathing).

Diagnosis

- Thoracic radiographs to diagnose ME and evaluate for aspiration pneumonia.
- Additional diagnostics for acquired ME:
  - Acetylcholine receptor antibody titers.
  - Blood lead concentration.
  - Resting cortisol concentration.
  - Thyroid testing (T_4, TSH, etc.).
  - Esophagoscopy.
  - Muscle biopsy.
  - Nerve conduction studies.
  - Swallow studies.

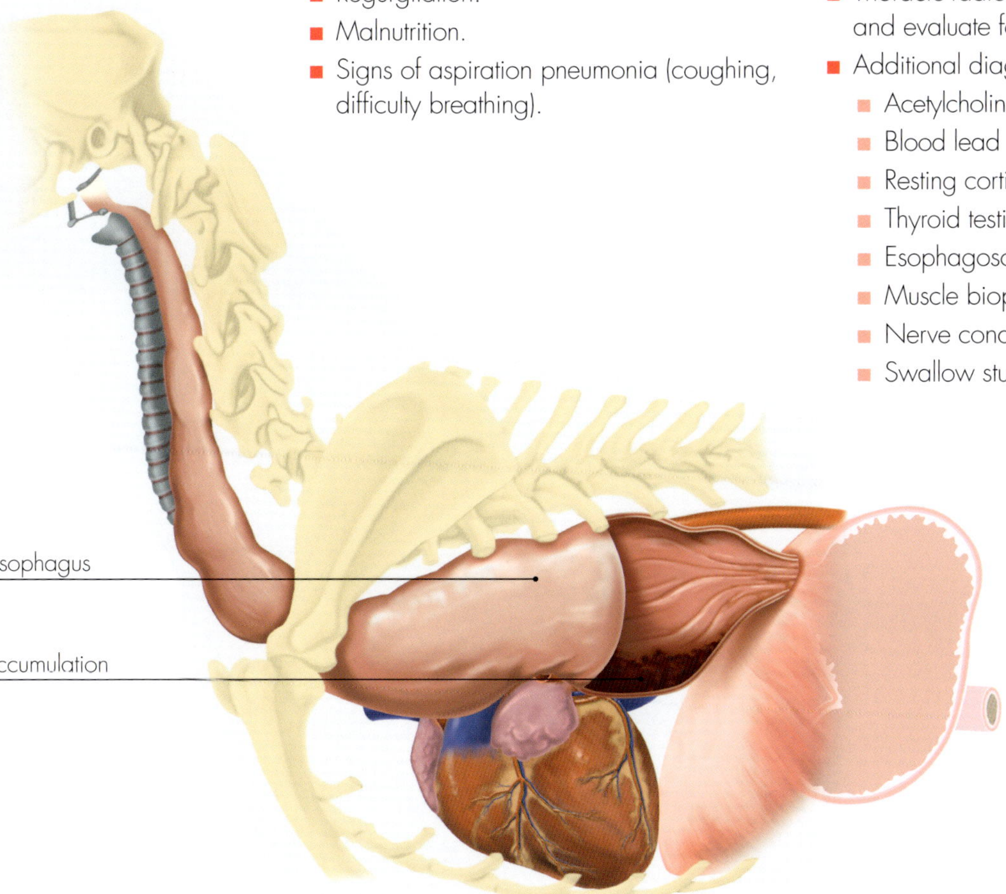

Treatment

- Treatment of the underlying cause of acquired ME.
- Medical management:
  - Upright feeding (e.g., Bailey chair) to utilize gravity to facilitate the passage of food into the stomach.
  - Vary the consistency of food (liquid, canned meatballs, kibble) to determine which is best tolerated.
  - Appropriate antibiotic therapy in case of aspiration pneumonia.
  - Sildenafil to relax the lower esophageal sphincter.
  - Cisapride may be useful in cats.

Prognosis

- Dogs with congenital or idiopathic acquired ME generally succumb to recurrent bouts of aspiration pneumonia.

Prokinetics such as cisapride and metoclopramide have no effect on esophageal striated muscle and will tighten the lower esophageal sphincter. Therefore, they generally should be avoided in dogs with ME.

DISEASES OF THE ESOPHAGUS

12 Hiatal hernia

A hiatal hernia occurs when the organs in the abdomen, most commonly the stomach, pass through a defect in the diaphragm and into the chest cavity. In most patients, hiatal hernias are congenital (birth) defects that occur secondary to incomplete fusion of the diaphragm during early development. Brachycephalic (short-nosed) dogs are at the highest risk of developing a hiatal hernia. Less commonly, acquired hiatal hernias can occur in any breed of cat or dog secondary to chronic increases in intra-abdominal pressure (e.g., chronic vomiting) or decreases in intrathoracic pressure (e.g., intermittent airway obstruction secondary to laryngeal paralysis).

Clinical signs

- Often no clinical signs.
- Regurgitation.
- Vomiting.
- Hypersalivation.
- Signs of aspiration pneumonia.

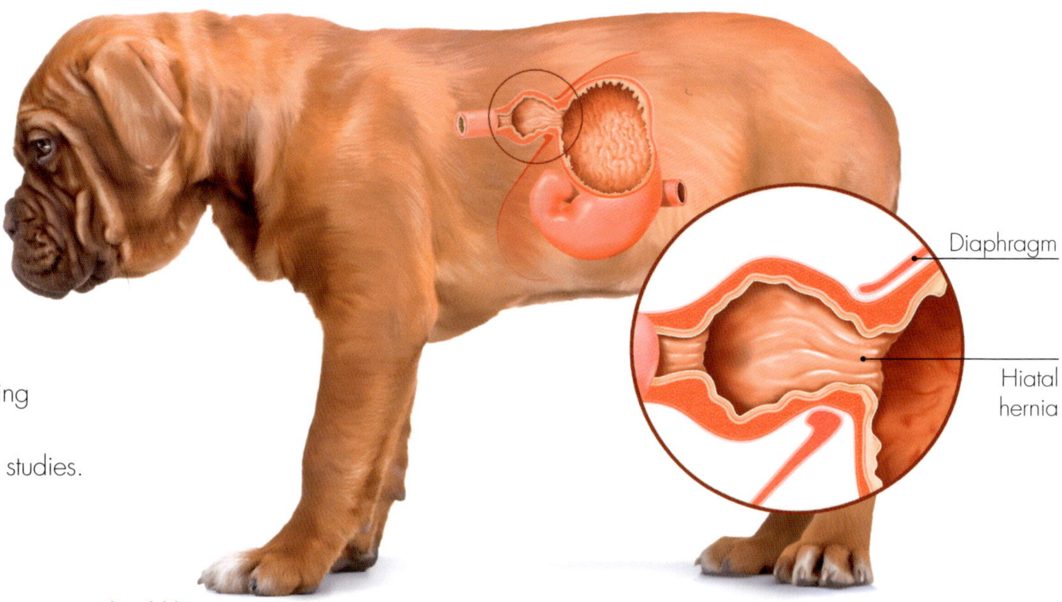

Diagnosis

- Radiographs (can miss sliding hiatal hernias).
- Videofluoroscopic swallow studies.
- Endoscopy.

Brachycephalic airway surgery should be performed to correct the negative pressure in the chest cavity. In many cases, this resolves the clinical signs of hiatal hernia.

Types of hiatal hernia

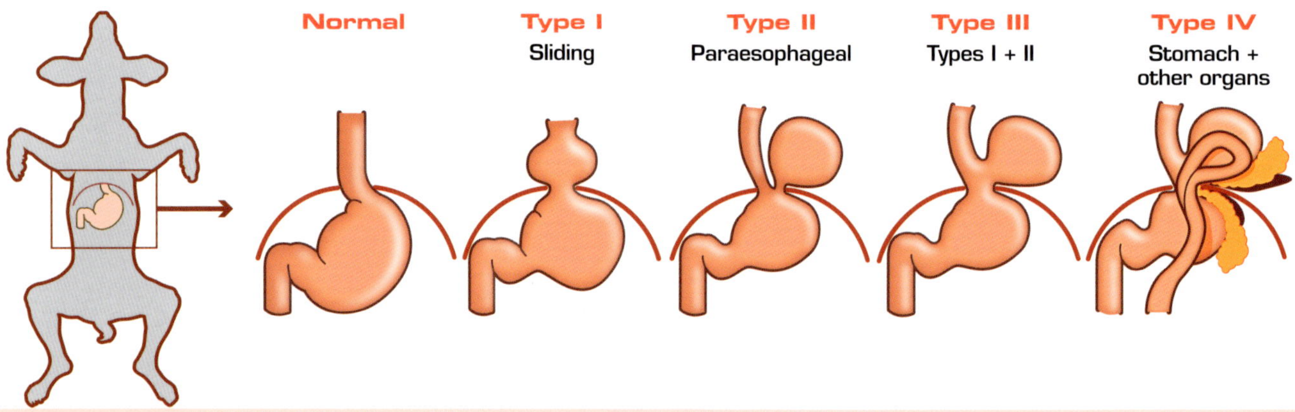

Treatment

- In cases without clinical signs, no treatment is necessary.
- Type I hiatal hernias may respond to conservative management for esophagitis (see Sheet 8).
- Surgery for clinical patients with a type II–IV hiatal hernia.

Prognosis

- Surgery may resolve the herniation and clinical signs.
- Dogs with clinical signs that do not undergo surgical correction are at risk of recurrent bouts of aspiration pneumonia.
- Bowel strangulation is possible.

DISEASES OF THE ESOPHAGUS

13 Gastroesophageal reflux

Gastroesophageal reflux is characterized by the backward flow of acidic gastric contents into the esophagus due to a weak lower esophageal sphincter. This is very irritating to the esophageal wall and results in esophagitis. Medications utilized for anesthesia can loosen the lower esophageal sphincter. Consequently, gastroesophageal reflux has been reported in 20%–50% of patients undergoing anesthetic events.

Preanesthetic administration of cisapride (with esomeprazole) or high-dose metoclopramide can reduce the incidence of anesthesia-induced acidic gastroesophageal reflux.

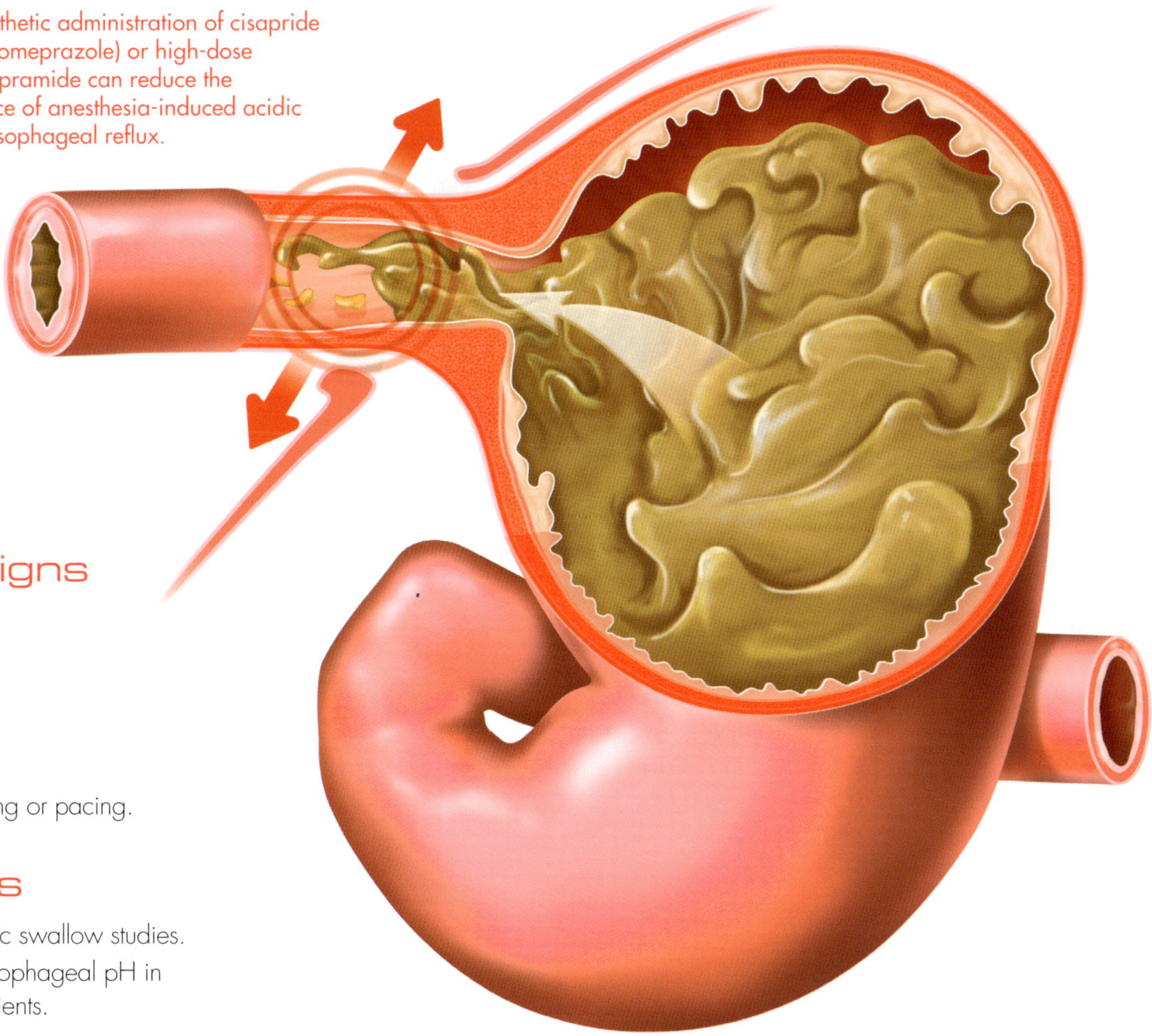

Clinical signs

- Regurgitation.
- Coughing.
- Gagging.
- Dysphagia.
- Voice change.
- Intermittent panting or pacing.

Diagnosis

- Videofluoroscopic swallow studies.
- Monitoring of esophageal pH in anesthetized patients.

Treatment

- Proton pump inhibitors (omeprazole) to decrease the acidity of gastric reflux fluids.
- Low-fat, low-fiber, canned food in small frequent meals to increase gastric emptying.
- Systemic analgesics for pain management.
- Cisapride (or metoclopramide) to increase lower esophageal sphincter tone.
- Aspiration of esophageal fluid and/or instillation of dilute bicarbonate solution if aspiration under general anesthesia is observed.

Prognosis

- Good if no complications arise.
- Anesthesia-induced gastroesophageal reflux has been associated with esophagitis, esophageal strictures, aspiration pneumonia, and nasopharyngeal stenosis.

DISEASES OF THE STOMACH

14 Acute gastritis

Acute gastritis is a syndrome commonly characterized by a sudden onset of vomiting due to gastric mucosal insult or inflammation. It can be caused by dietary indiscretion, foreign bodies, drugs/toxins (e.g., NSAIDs, antibiotics, chemotherapeutics), or infectious diseases. In some cases, the cause is inferred from the history.

Clinical signs

- Vomiting (acute onset).
- Possible additional signs:
  - Hematemesis, melena.
  - Signs of systemic illness.

Diagnosis

- Usually based on clinical findings and response to symptomatic treatment.
- History (medication history, toxin exposure, dietary indiscretion, foreign body ingestion).
- Abdominal radiographs.
- Complete blood count and chemistry profile (to evaluate for systemic causes of vomiting) ± canine pancreatic lipase immunoreactivity.
- Testing for gastric parasites.

Abdominal radiographs should be performed in all patients with acute vomiting of unknown cause.

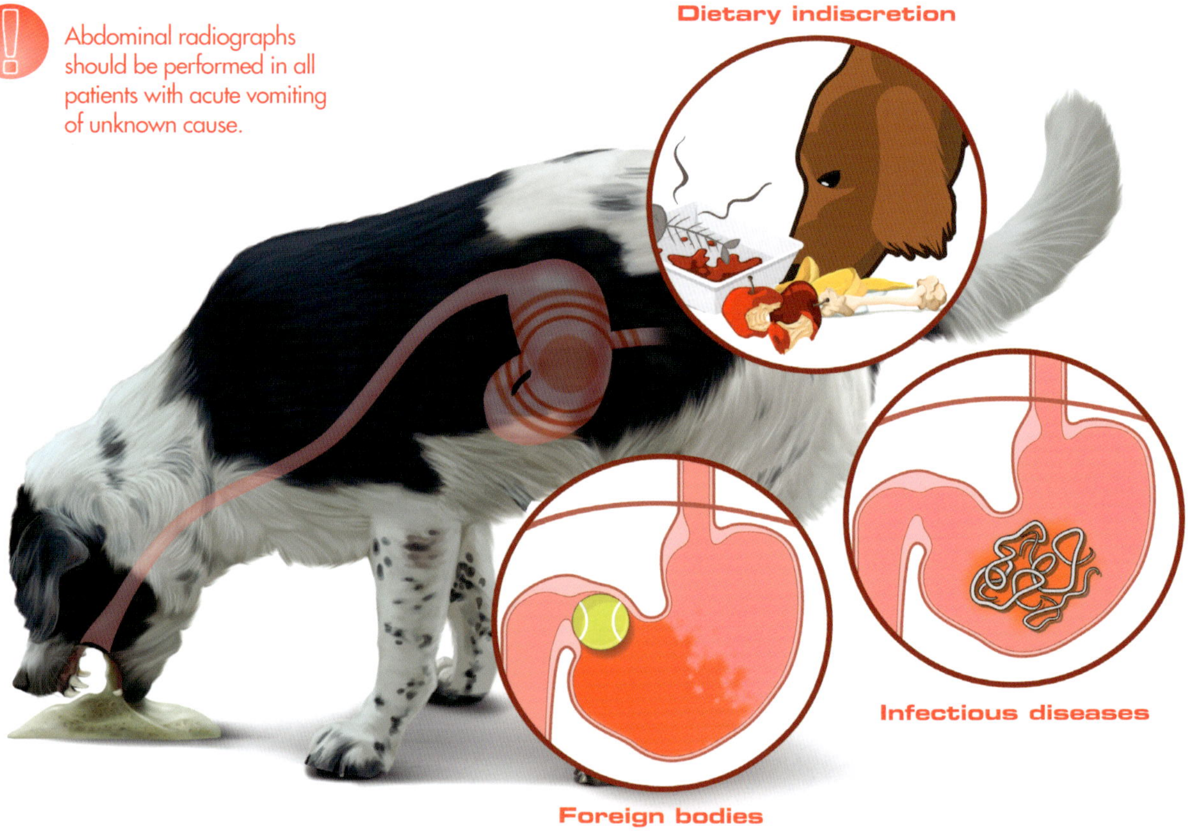

Treatment

- Fluid therapy to address dehydration (small frequent amounts orally, subcutaneously, or intravenously). Pets requiring intravenous fluids warrant a more extensive diagnostic evaluation.
- Withhold food for 12–24 hours and then introduce small amounts of a low-fat, bland diet (e.g., boiled chicken and rice, commercial diet).
- Antiemetics (maropitant, ondansetron) for 2–3 days after ruling out obstruction.
- Protectants/absorbents (bismuth subsalicylate, kaolin–pectin, sucralfate, barium).
- Proton pump inhibitors (omeprazole) if hematemesis or melena are present.
- Treatment of underlying causes if present.

Prognosis

- Good to excellent for complete recovery of uncomplicated acute gastritis.

DISEASES OF THE STOMACH

15 Chronic gastritis

Gastritis that returns or remains unresolved (>2 weeks) with symptomatic treatment is classified as chronic gastritis. In the absence of systemic disease, drugs, toxins, gastric foreign material, parasites (*Physaloptera*, *Ollulanus*), cancer, or fungal infections (*Pythium insidiosum*, *Histoplasma*), chronic gastritis is usually attributed to dietary intolerance or allergy, occult parasitism, *Helicobacter* infection, or unknown pathogens. Chronic gastritis is thought to develop from the interplay between pathogens, the microbiota, and the immune system.

Clinical signs

- Vomiting (chronic).
- Possible additional signs:
  - Decreased appetite.
  - Weight loss.
  - Hematemesis, melena.

35% of dogs investigated for chronic vomiting have chronic gastritis.

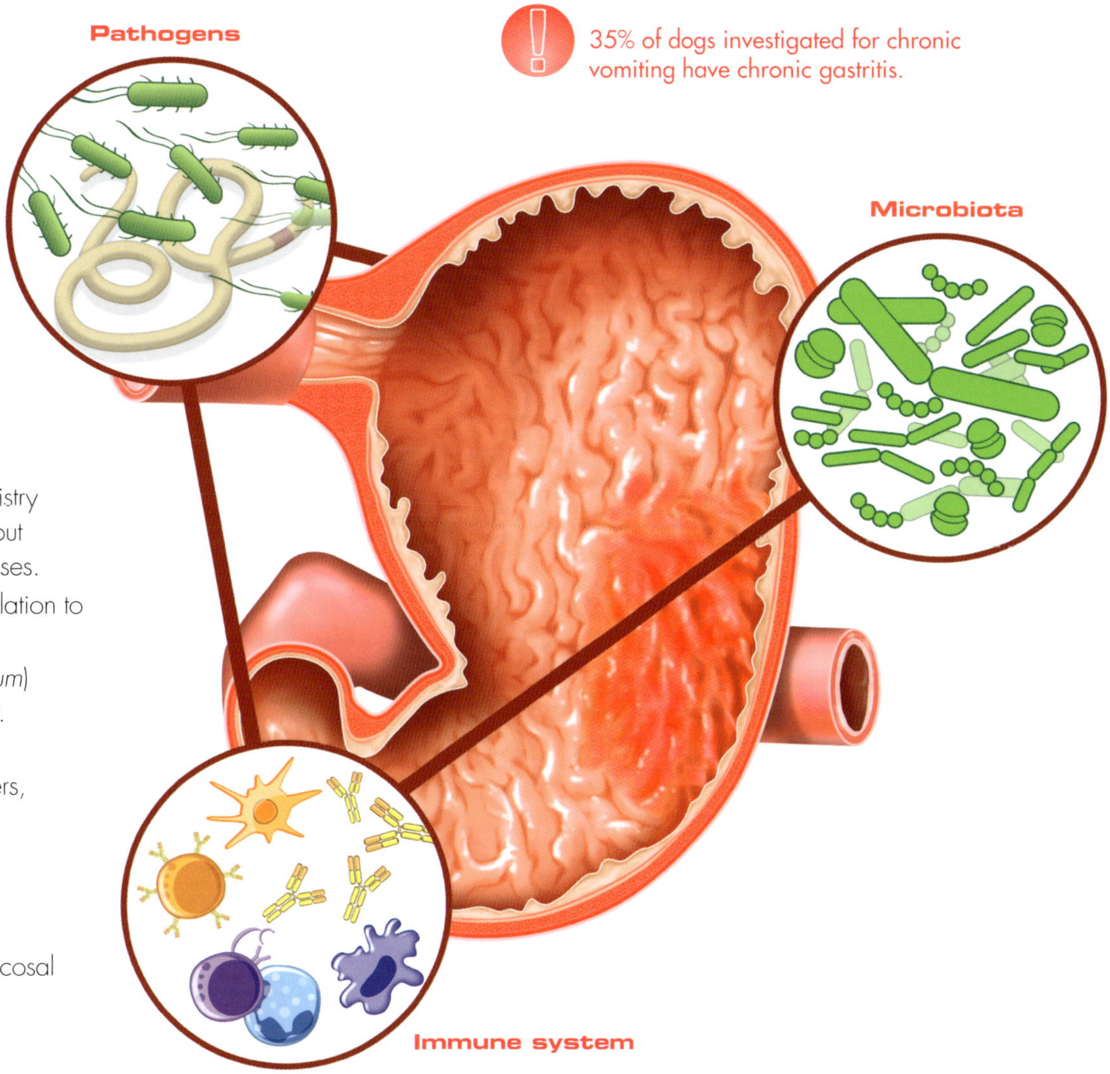

Diagnosis

- Complete blood count, chemistry profile, and urinalysis to rule out metabolic and endocrine causes.
- Resting cortisol ± ACTH stimulation to rule out hypoadrenocorticism.
- Infectious disease (e.g., *Pythium*) testing based on travel history.
- Abdominal radiographs and ultrasound to evaluate for ulcers, gastric wall thickening, and lymphadenopathy.
- Endoscopy and biopsy.
- Serum gastrin if unexplained gastric erosions, ulcers, or mucosal hypertrophy are found.

Treatment

- Empirical deworming (fenbendazole) and a hypoallergenic (hydrolyzed, novel protein) diet trial.
- Proton pump inhibitors and gastroprotectants if hematemesis or melena are present.
- If *Helicobacter*-associated gastritis is suspected, other more likely causes should be ruled out before considering treatment.
- Immunosuppressive therapy (prednisone) can be considered after ruling out other causes.

Prognosis

- Fungal or algal gastritis may carry a poor prognosis.
- *Helicobacter*-associated gastritis may require longer treatment durations.

DISEASES OF THE STOMACH

16 Gastric dilatation and volvulus (GDV)

GDV is a rapidly progressive, life-threatening condition in which the stomach becomes dramatically distended with air and twists upon itself such that both the entrance and exit to the stomach become closed off. The dilated stomach compresses nearby vessels, preventing adequate blood return to the heart. The stomach is at increased risk of tissue death (due to lack of blood flow) and rupture. Large-breed dogs with deep chests, such as the Great Dane, are at a greater risk for GDV.

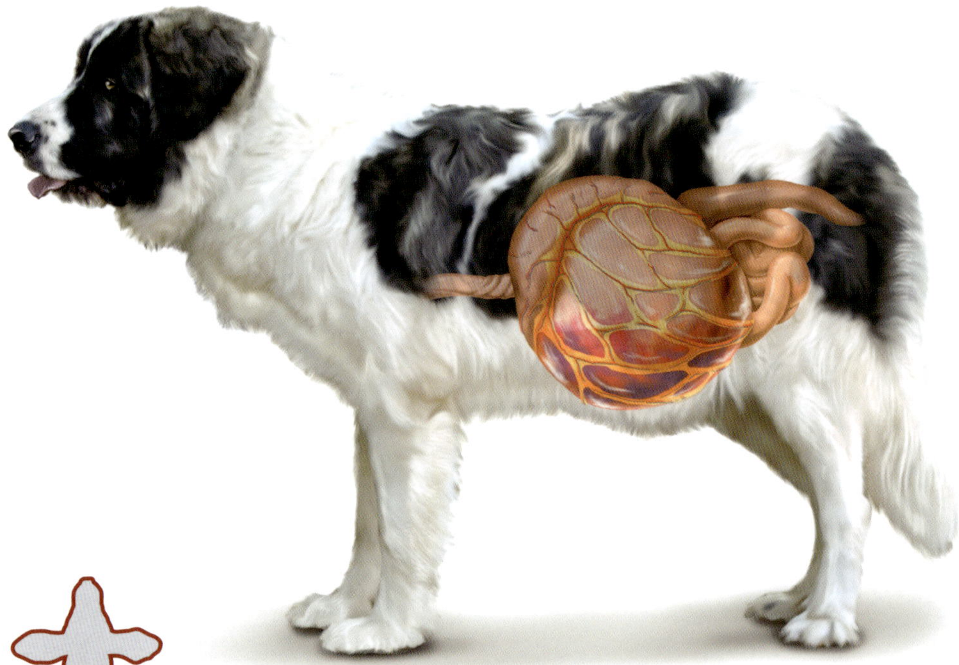

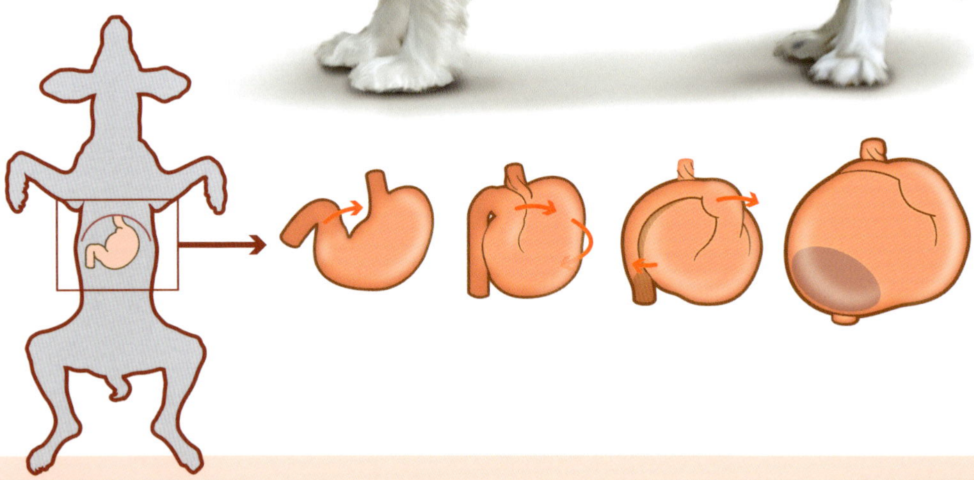

Clinical signs

- Nonproductive retching.
- Abdominal distension.
- Hypersalivation.
- Anxious pacing.
- Weakness, collapse.

Diagnosis

- Abdominal radiographs (right lateral): pylorus dorsal and cranial to the fundus (depends on degree of rotation).
- Complete blood count and chemistry profile with a blood gas test to evaluate for metabolic disturbances.
- Electrocardiogram to evaluate for arrhythmias.

! GDV is considered a surgical emergency.

Treatment

- Stabilization prior to surgery is essential:
  - Intravenous fluids to restore circulating blood volume.
  - Oxygen therapy to support the respiratory system.
  - Gastric decompression to relieve pressure and prevent tissue damage.
- Surgery:
  - Determine the viability of the stomach wall, spleen, and other organs.
  - Derotate stomach ± gastric resection ± splenectomy.
  - Gastropexy (stomach fixed to the abdominal wall to prevent rotation).

Prognosis

- Mortality rate: 10%–15%; higher (>30%) in dogs that have gastric resection, gastric necrosis, splenectomy, longer times from presentation to surgery, or arrhythmias.
- Gastric dilatation can reoccur, but the gastropexy will prevent a life-threatening volvulus.
- Prophylactic gastropexy in high-risk breeds can reduce mortality.

DISEASES OF THE STOMACH

17 Delayed gastric emptying

Delayed gastric emptying is the most common disorder of gastric motility. It is a consequence of conditions that either result in defective propulsion or create an outflow obstruction. Defective propulsion can result from gastritis, gastric dilatation and volvulus, gastric ulcers, gastric cancer, pancreatitis, surgery, hospitalization, drugs (anticholinergics, narcotics), electrolyte derangements (hypokalemia, hypocalcemia), metabolic disorders (hypoadrenocorticism, uremia), peritonitis, or pain. Outflow obstruction–induced delayed gastric emptying is caused by any mechanical obstruction (e.g., foreign bodies, polyps, cancer, congenital stenosis, hypertrophy of the pyloric mucosa).

Clinical signs

- Vomiting (>8 hours after ingestion).
- Possible additional signs:
  - Weight loss.
  - Abdominal discomfort, bloating.

Diagnosis

- Barium contrast studies to document delayed gastric emptying time.
- Abdominal radiographs and ultrasound to screen for extragastric disorders (e.g., pancreatitis).
- Endoscopy and biopsy.

Normal pylorus

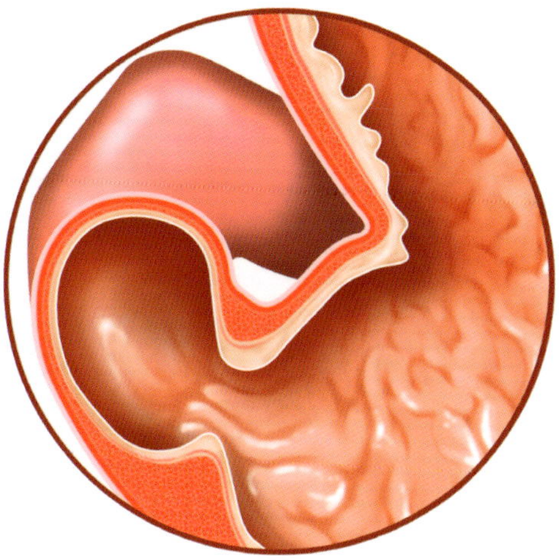

Pyloric stenosis

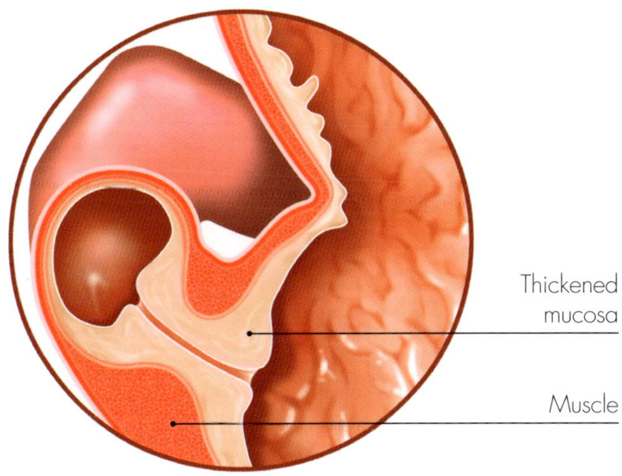

Normal gastric emptying

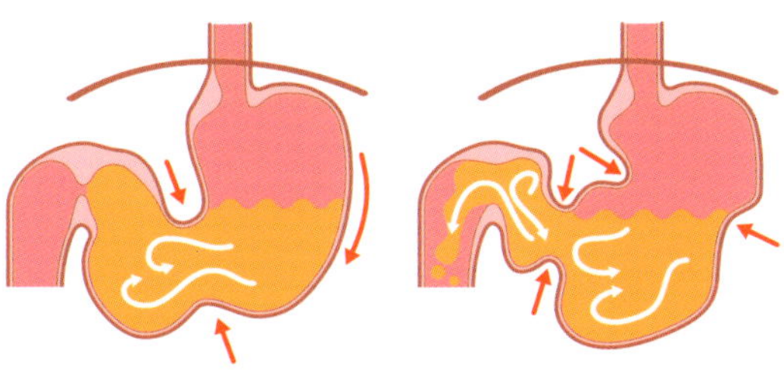

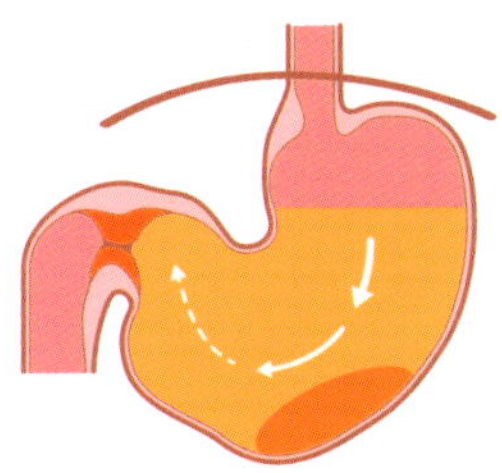

Delayed gastric emptying

Treatment

- Treatment of underlying causes:
  - Treatment of gastroduodenal ulcers (see Sheet 18).
  - Endoscopy or surgery in case of foreign body (see Sheet 34).
  - Surgery in case of pyloric stenosis or polyps.
- Medical management for disorders of defective propulsion:
  - Low-fat, low-fiber, canned diet in small frequent meals.
  - Prokinetics (cisapride, metoclopramide, ranitidine).

Prognosis

- Dependent on the underlying cause.

DISEASES OF THE STOMACH

18 Gastroduodenal ulcers

A gastroduodenal ulcer is a defect in the wall of the stomach or duodenum that extends through the muscularis mucosa into the deeper layers (submucosa) of the gastric or intestinal wall. Given the presence of vessels in these deeper tissues, life-threatening hemorrhage may result. With severe ulceration, perforation of the wall may occur, resulting in bacterial contamination of the abdominal cavity. The most common causes of ulceration are drug-associated injuries (NSAIDs), mast cell tumors, and primary gastric and duodenal tumors. Sled dogs may suffer from exercise-induced gastroduodenal ulcers. Gastrinomas, a tumor of the pancreas which produces the hormone gastrin, may result in ulcer formation, but mucosal hypertrophy and delayed gastric emptying are more commonly detected.

Clinical signs

- Vomiting.
- Hematemesis, melena.
- Abdominal pain.
- Weight loss.

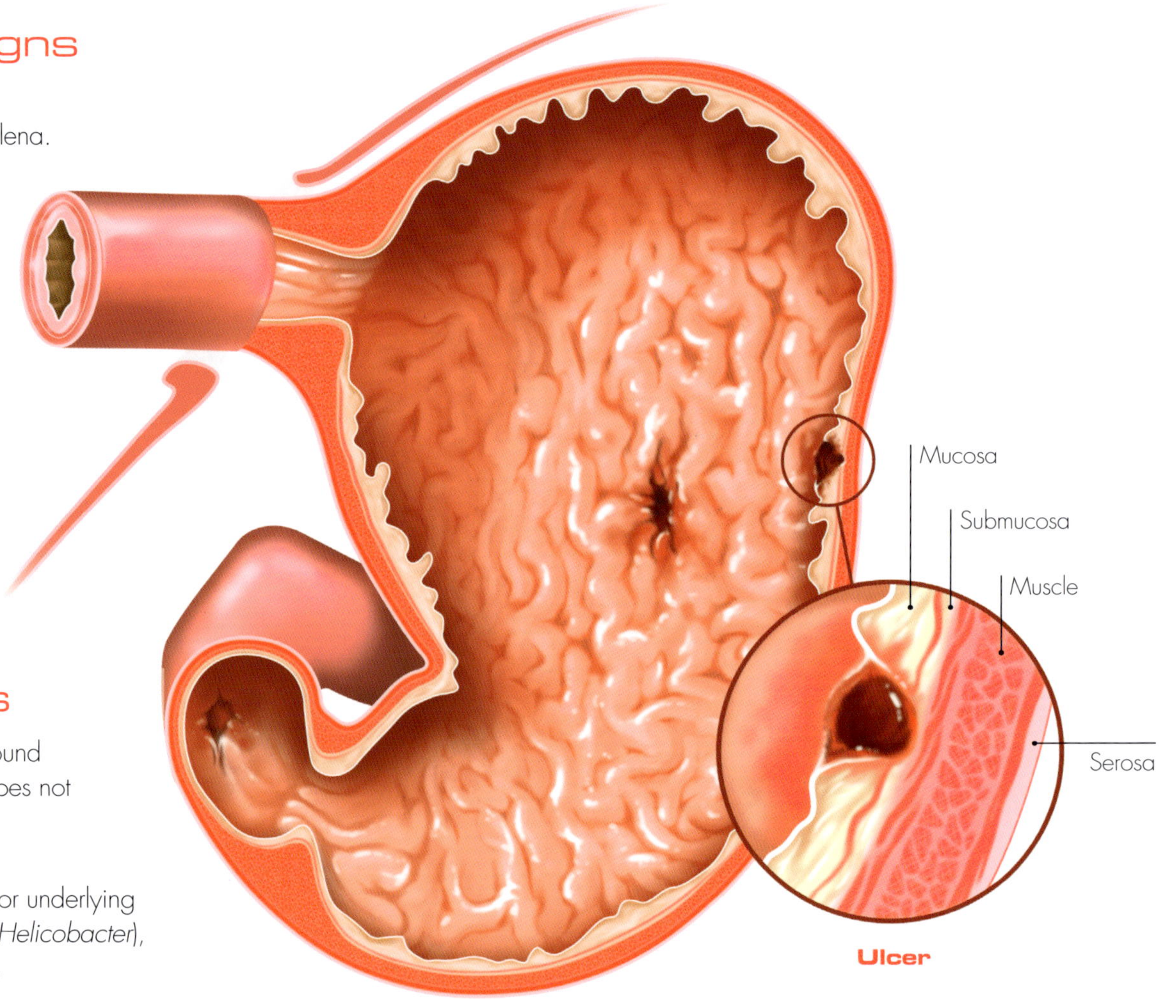

Diagnosis

- Abdominal ultrasound (a normal study does not rule out ulcers).
- Endoscopy.
- Biopsy to screen for underlying cancer, infection (*Helicobacter*), and inflammation.

Treatment

- Treatment of underlying causes when possible.
- Sucralfate slurry to protect the gastric mucosa.
- Proton pump inhibitors (omeprazole) to decrease the acidity of gastric fluid.
- Low-fat, low-fiber, canned food in small frequent meals.
- Systemic analgesics for pain management.
- Surgical resection of ulcers that are refractory to medical management or have perforated.

Prognosis

- Dependent on the underlying cause, severity of the clinical signs, and whether or not perforation has occurred.

DISEASES OF THE SMALL INTESTINE

19 Acute enteritis

Acute enteritis is a syndrome characterized by the sudden onset of diarrhea and/or vomiting caused by gastrointestinal mucosal inflammation. There are many causes of acute enteritis including dietary indiscretion, toxin ingestion, foreign body ingestion, parasites, viral infections, bacterial infections, intussusceptions, and acute pancreatitis.

Clinical signs

- Vomiting.
- Diarrhea.
- Hematemesis, melena.
- Abdominal pain.
- Decreased appetite.

Diagnosis

- Usually based on clinical findings and response to symptomatic treatment.
- History (medication history, toxin exposure, dietary indiscretion, foreign body ingestion).
- Further diagnostics are indicated if the patient is dull, depressed, febrile, dehydrated, or has abdominal pain.

Most cases of acute enteritis are self-limiting. If clinical signs persist beyond 3 days, further diagnostics are warranted.

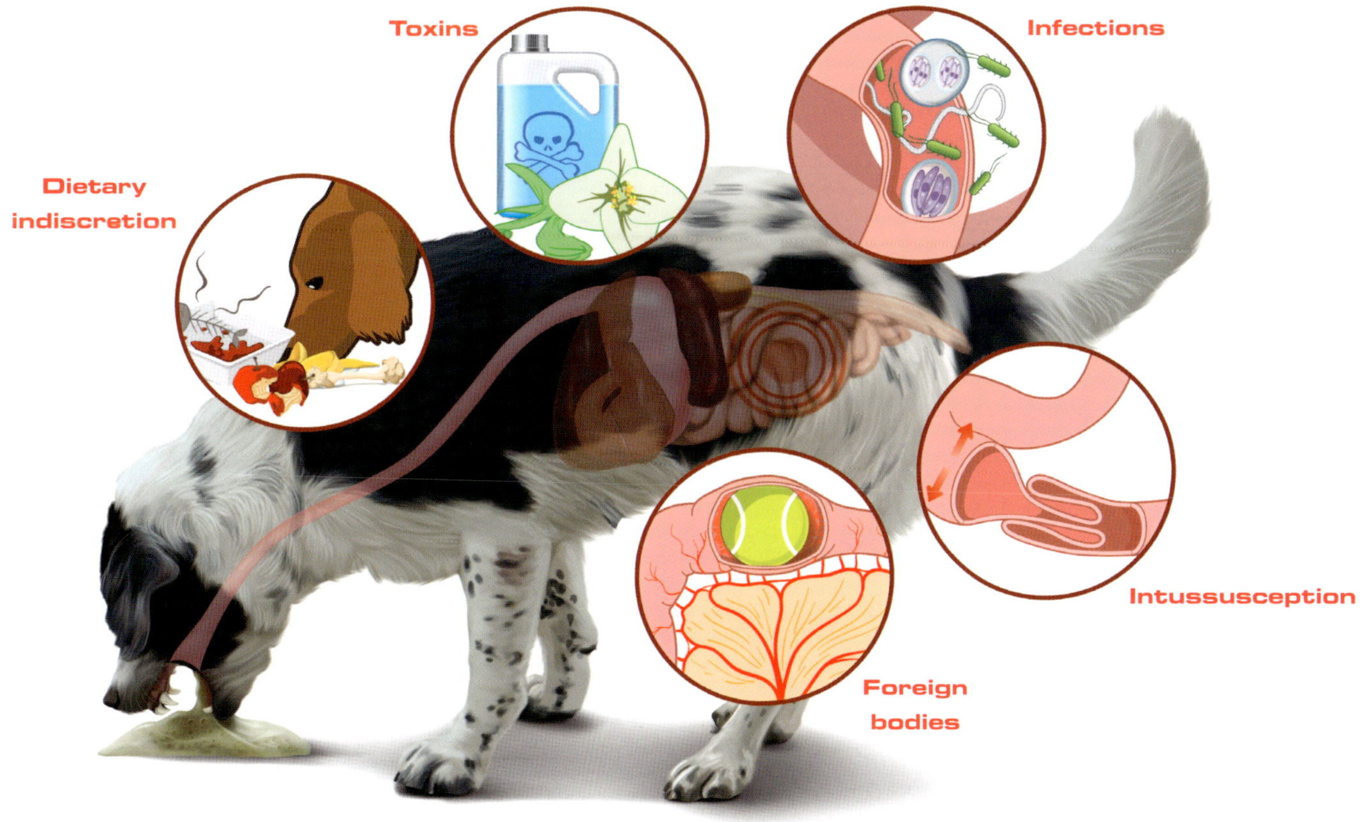

Treatment

- Fluid therapy.
- Management of vomiting (see Sheet 14).
- Management of diarrhea:
  - Easily digestible diets. Fiber-containing diets for large bowel diarrhea.
  - Probiotics can be considered.
  - Antidiarrheal therapy (loperamide, metronidazole) is often not needed.
- Antibiotics should be reserved for cases with suspected sepsis.
- Treatment of underlying causes if present.

Prognosis

- Good to excellent for complete recovery in uncomplicated cases of acute enteritis.

DISEASES OF THE SMALL INTESTINE

20 Acute hemorrhagic diarrheal syndrome (AHDS)

AHDS, formally known as hemorrhagic gastroenteritis, is a syndrome in dogs characterized by acute vomiting and hemorrhagic diarrhea, often accompanied by hemoconcentration. Although any dog can be affected, young (median age 4 years old) small-breed dogs are overrepresented. The cause remains unknown, but the bacterium *Clostridium perfringens* may be involved.

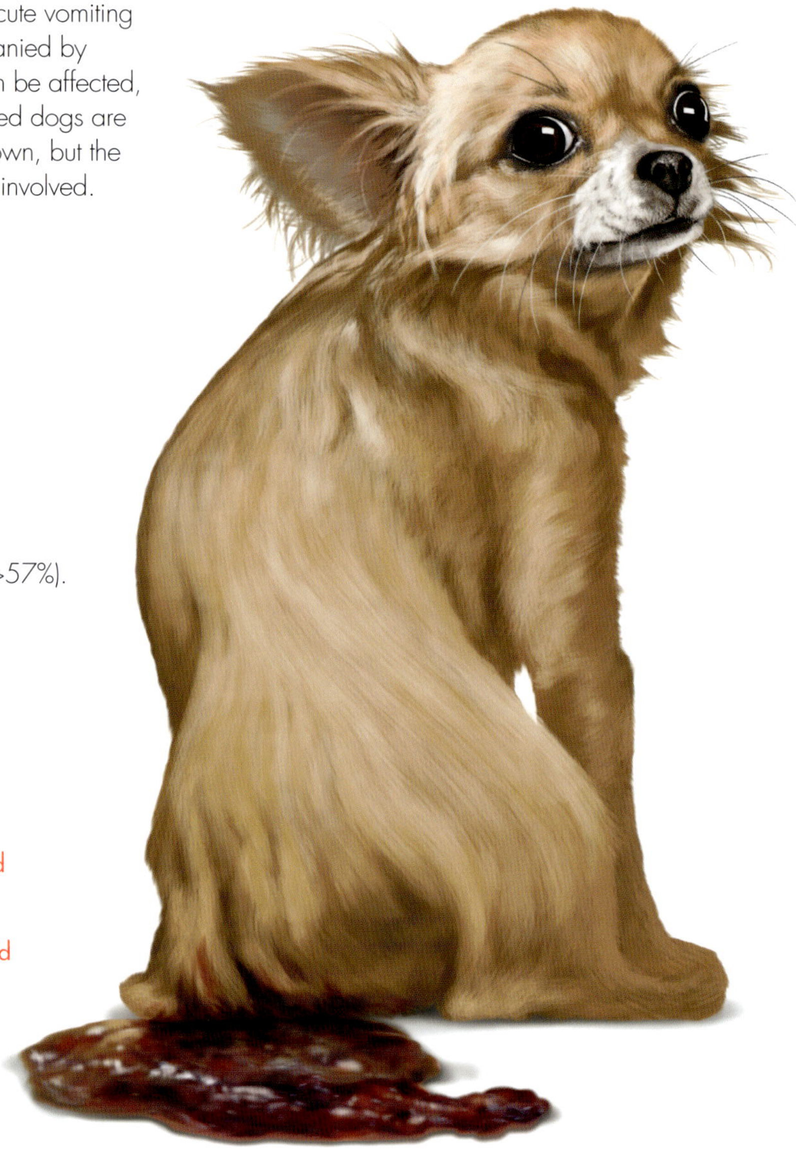

Clinical signs

- Vomiting (often first clinical sign).
- Watery, bloody diarrhea.
- Dehydration.

Diagnosis

- Acute onset of hemorrhagic diarrhea.
- Severe hemoconcentration (hematocrit >57%).
- Relatively low serum total protein.
- Rapid response to intravenous fluids.

The finding of hemoconcentration and a relatively low serum total protein concentration in an adult small-breed dog with hemorrhagic diarrhea should increase suspicion of AHDS.

Treatment

- Intravenous fluid therapy.
- Symptomatic treatment of vomiting (anti-nausea medications) and diarrhea.
- Nutritional support.
- Antibiotics should be reserved for cases with suspected sepsis.

Prognosis

- Good with early and appropriate treatment.
- Without treatment, severe dehydration, hypovolemia, and death may occur.

DISEASES OF THE SMALL INTESTINE

21 Canine parvovirus infection

Canine parvovirus is a highly contagious virus that can affect all dogs, but unvaccinated dogs and puppies (<4 months) are at the greatest risk. Following fecal–oral transmission, canine parvovirus 2 (CPV-2) invades and destroys rapidly dividing cells (e.g., intestinal crypt epithelium, bone marrow progenitors), producing severe gastrointestinal signs and neutropenia. Viral infection of the intestinal crypt cells leads to cell death and loss of the normal barrier function, resulting in translocation of bacteria. Parvovirus-induced gastrointestinal signs can lead to devastating and life-threatening fluid and electrolyte losses.

CPV-2 is hardy and may persist in the environment for long periods of time (5–7 months).

Clinical signs

- Depression, anorexia.
- Severe diarrhea and vomiting (24–48 hours after illness onset).
- Fever.
- Abdominal pain.
- Systemic inflammatory response syndrome (SIRS).

Diagnosis

- Neutropenia in a puppy with severe gastrointestinal signs is suggestive but not diagnostic.
- Fecal parvovirus antigen enzyme linked immunosorbent assay (ELISA).

Dogs with parvovirus enteritis may develop intussusception. Therefore, they should undergo regular abdominal palpation.

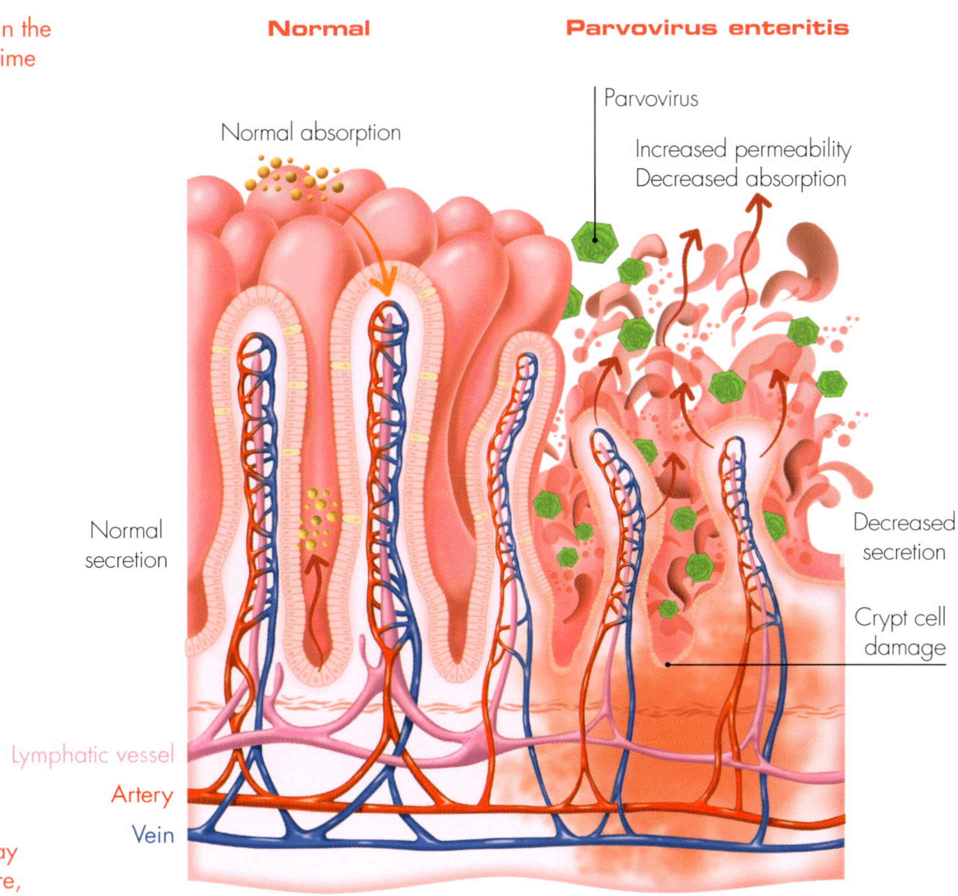

Treatment

- Aggressive intravenous fluid therapy: crystalloids ± colloids (fresh frozen plasma, hydroxyethyl starch).
- Antiemetics for vomiting.
- Broad-spectrum antibiotics: penicillins, fluroquinolones, aminoglycosides (in euhydrated patients). Enrofloxacin should be avoided in young large-breed dogs due to cartilage damage.
- Prompt enteral nutrition.
- Analgesia.
- Frequent monitoring of hydration status, electrolytes, hematocrit, serum proteins, and blood glucose.
- Fecal microbiota transplantation.

Prognosis

- Mortality rate in treated dogs: 4%–48%.
- Negative prognostic indicators: leukopenia, neutropenia, lymphopenia, SIRS at presentation, hypoalbuminemia.
- Without treatment, severe dehydration, hypovolemia, and death (91% mortality rate) occur.

DISEASES OF THE SMALL INTESTINE

22 Intestinal dysbiosis

An estimated trillion microbes live within the gastrointestinal tract. The decrease in diversity or richness of these microbes is known as dysbiosis. Dysbiosis is associated with a number of disorders of the gastrointestinal tract, including chronic enteropathies, acute hemorrhagic diarrheal syndrome, acute enteritis, exocrine pancreatic insufficiency, intestinal stasis (cancer, foreign bodies), and motility disorders, as well as with the administration of antibiotics.

Clinical signs

- Intermittent chronic diarrhea.
- Weight loss.
- Other clinical signs due to the primary underlying disorder.

Diagnosis

- Dysbiosis index if available.
- High serum folate and low serum cobalamin concentrations.

In one study of dogs with small intestinal dysbiosis, only 50% had an increased serum folate concentration and only 35% had a decreased serum cobalamin concentration.

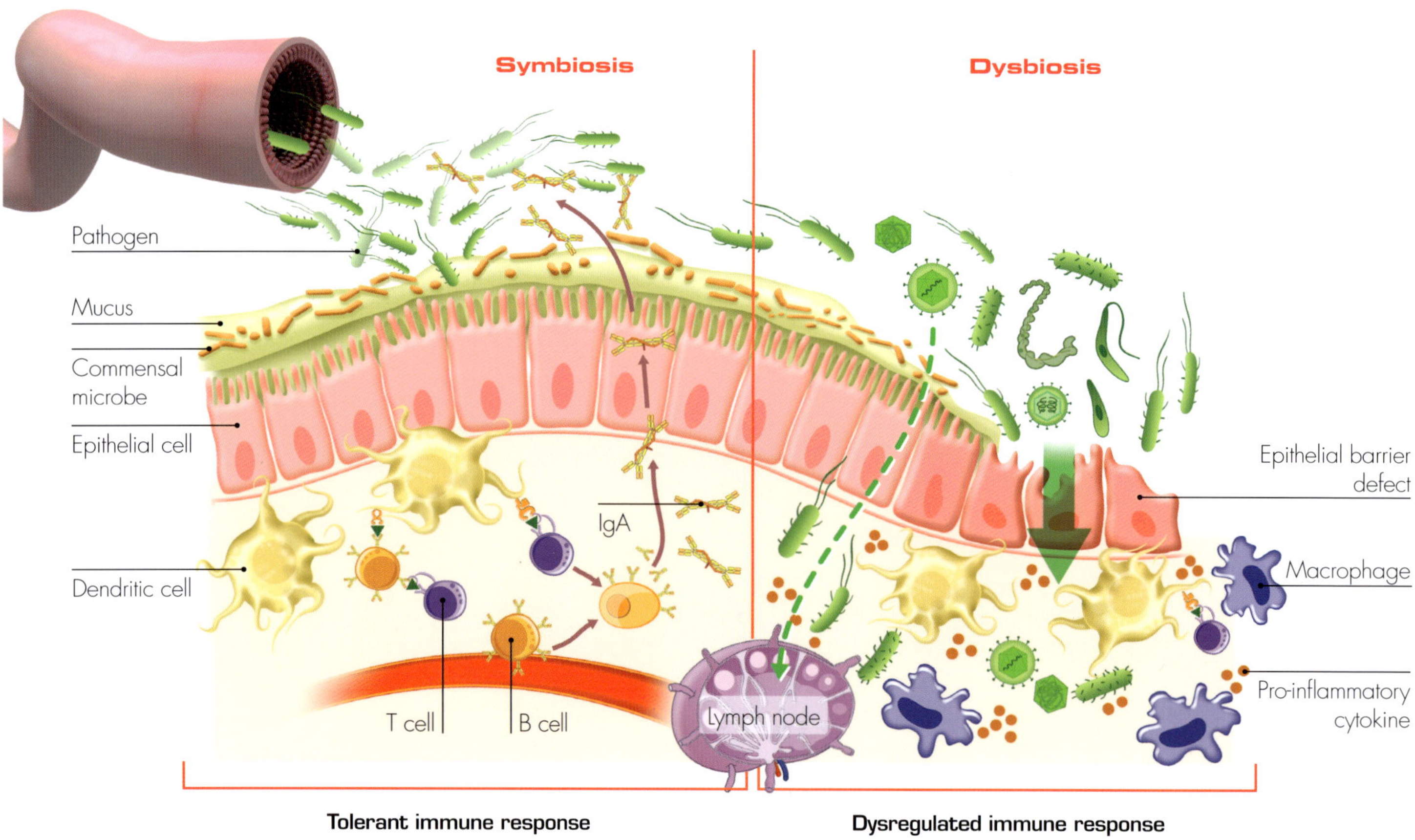

Treatment

- Treatment of the inciting cause (e.g., exocrine pancreatic insufficiency, chronic enteropathy).
- Probiotics.
- Fecal microbiota transplantation (see Sheet 44).
- Antibiotics (tylosin, metronidazole) after ruling out other conditions and if supported by diagnostics.

Prognosis

- Largely dependent on the underlying cause.

DISEASES OF THE SMALL INTESTINE

23 Chronic enteropathy

Chronic enteropathy (CE) is an umbrella term relating to a host of diseases characterized by gastrointestinal signs that persist for at least 3 weeks. Although inflammatory bowel disease (IBD) is a form of CE, the diagnosis of IBD requires a systematic therapeutic approach to rule out food-responsive, fiber-responsive, and antibiotic-responsive disease. By following this approach, many dogs and cats with CE can be successfully treated before undergoing invasive and costly endoscopic procedures.

Clinical signs

- Any combination of gastrointestinal clinical signs (e.g., vomiting, diarrhea, weight loss, changes in appetite) present for more than 3 weeks.

Diagnosis

- Exclusion of extragastrointestinal diseases:
  - Complete blood count, chemistry profile, urinalysis, and abdominal imaging.
  - Trypsin-like immunoreactivity.
  - Resting cortisol.
  - Total T_4 in cats.
- Geographically relevant infectious disease testing.
- Fecal parasite testing.
- Serum cobalamin and folate to screen for malabsorption.
- Response to therapy (see below).
- Endoscopy if there is no response to therapy.

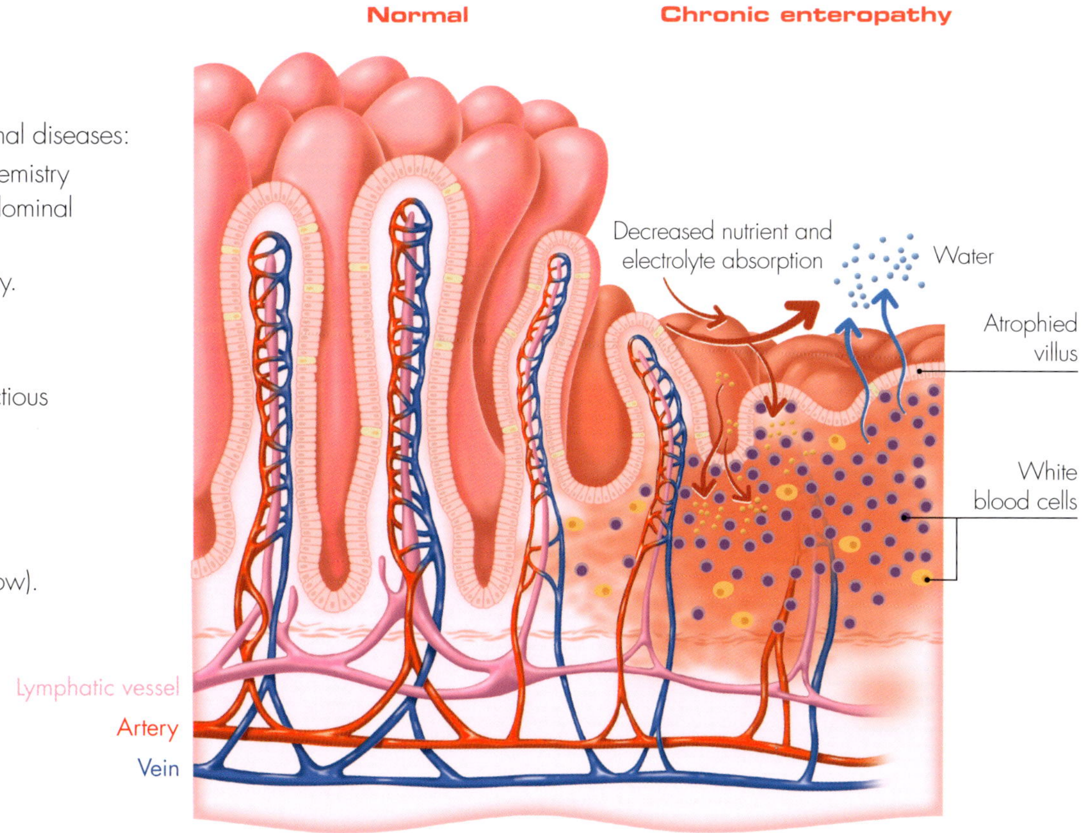

Treatment

- Empirical deworming to rule out parasitic disease.
- Diet trials: fed exclusively (no treats, flavored medications, or oral preventatives) for 2–3 weeks.
  - Easily digestible low-fat diet.
  - Fiber-rich diet if large bowel diarrhea.
  - Novel protein, limited ingredient, or hydrolyzed diets if there is no response to easily digestible diets.
- Probiotic and antibiotic (tylosin, metronidazole) trials.
- After the histopathologic diagnosis of lymphoplasmacytic ± eosinophilic enteritis and treating for parasitism and antibiotic- and food-responsive disease, corticosteroids for the treatment of idiopathic CE.

Prognosis

- Variable and largely dependent on the underlying cause.

DISEASES OF THE SMALL INTESTINE

24 Intestinal lymphangiectasia

Intestinal lymphangiectasia is a disease of the intestinal lymphatic system in dogs. This enteropathy results in the loss of proteins, predominately albumin, via the gastrointestinal tract. Loss of globulin and cholesterol may also be seen. When albumin loss through the gastrointestinal tract is severe (serum albumin <1.8 g/dl), effusion (loss of fluid into a body cavity) or edema may occur. Dogs with intestinal lymphangiectasia may also be hypercoagulable from enteric loss of antithrombin, or hypocalcemic from poor absorption of vitamin D. Although primary intestinal lymphangiectasia is most common, it may occur secondary to inflammatory bowel disease, cancer, or infectious disease.

Intestinal lymphangiectasia can occur in any dog, but Yorkshire Terriers, Soft-Coated Wheaten Terriers, and Norwegian Lundehunds appear to be at a greater risk.

Clinical signs

- Small bowel diarrhea.
- Weight loss, typically despite a good appetite.
- Vomiting.
- Abdominal or pleural effusion.
- Edema.

Diagnosis

- Documentation of hypoalbuminemia or panhypoproteinemia with hypocholesterolemia.
- Resting cortisol to rule out hypoadrenocorticism.
- Urine protein:creatinine ratio to rule out protein-losing nephropathy.
- Bile acids to evaluate liver function.
- Abdominal ultrasound may reveal hyperechoic mucosal striations.
- Endoscopy and intestinal biopsy.

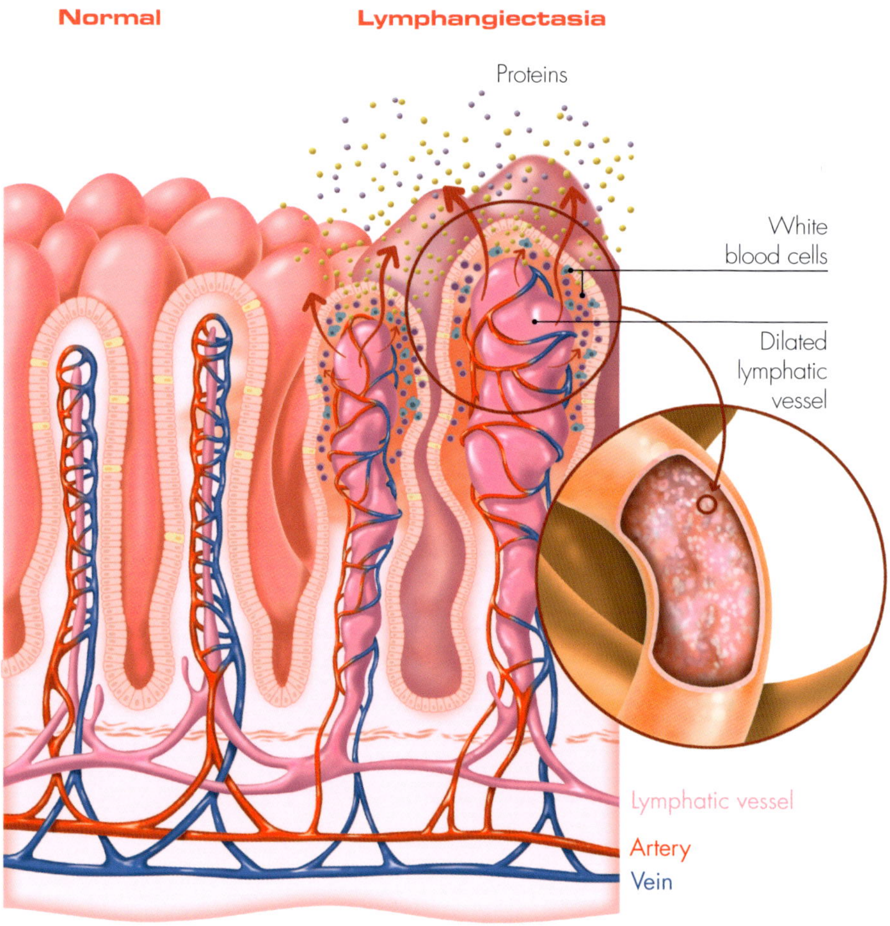

Treatment

- Treatment of underlying disease if present.
- Low-fat to ultra-low-fat diet.
- Antiplatelet drugs (e.g., clopidogrel) when evidence of thrombosis.
- Corticosteroids and other immunosuppressive therapy may be needed.

Prognosis

- Some dogs respond well to low-fat diets, while others require concurrent immunosuppressive therapy.
- Some dogs die despite dietary and immunosuppressive therapy.

DISEASES OF THE SMALL INTESTINE

25 Feline inflammatory bowel disease vs. small-cell lymphoma

The two major considerations in middle-aged to older cats with chronic gastrointestinal signs are inflammatory bowel disease (IBD) and small-cell lymphoma (SCL). The diagnostic and therapeutic approach to feline IBD follows that of chronic enteropathy to evaluate for food-responsive, parasitic, and steroid-responsive enteropathies. Biopsy is necessary for a diagnosis of SCL.

Clinical signs

- Vomiting.
- Diarrhea.
- Changes in appetite.
- Weight loss.

Diagnosis

- Total T_4 to screen for hyperthyroidism.
- FeLV and FIV testing.
- Fecal parasite testing.
- Abdominal ultrasound.
- Serum cobalamin and folate.
- Biopsy ± PARR:
  - Ideally samples from duodenum and ileum.
  - Full-thickness intestinal samples may be needed.

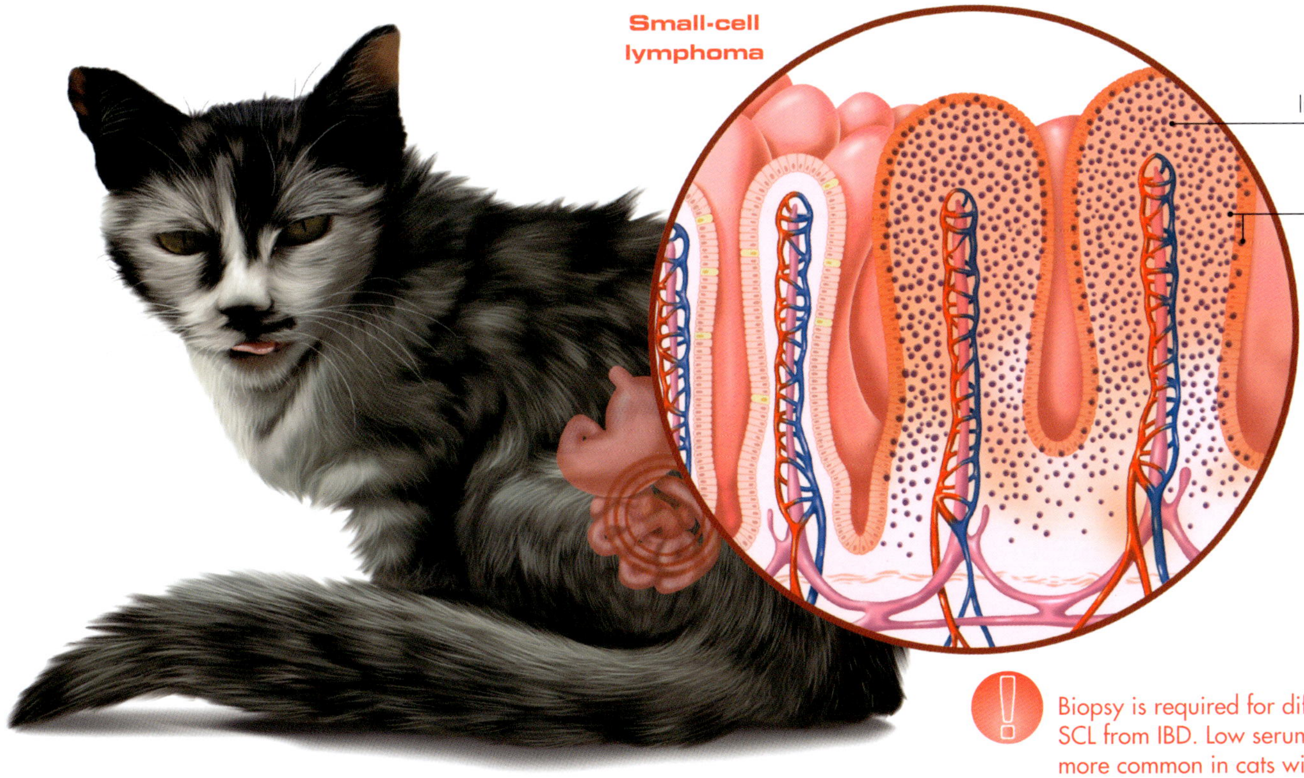

Biopsy is required for differentiating SCL from IBD. Low serum albumin is more common in cats with SCL.

Treatment

IBD

- Treatment of chronic enteropathy (see Sheet 23).
- Diet, deworming, probiotics, ± corticosteroids.

SCL

- Prednisolone and chlorambucil.

Prognosis

IBD

- Dependent on the underlying cause, but generally good.

SCL

- Good, with a median survival time of 2 years.
- 92% of cats respond to the combination therapy of prednisolone and chlorambucil.

DISEASES OF THE LARGE INTESTINE

26 Acute colitis

Acute colitis is a syndrome characterized by a sudden onset of diarrhea associated with the characteristic clinical signs of large bowel inflammation (i.e., increased urgency, small frequent volumes of stool, presence of mucus, hematochezia). Acute colitis typically follows dietary indiscretion, endoparasite infections (whipworms), or stress (recent boarding, grooming), although the exact cause is rarely identified. Traumatic acute colitis can be caused by the inappropriate ingestion of bones or other sharp indigestible objects. As most cases are self-limiting, management of acute colitis is largely supportive.

Clinical signs

- Acute onset of large bowel diarrhea.
- Possible additional signs:
  - Hematochezia.
  - Vomiting.

The finding of abdominal pain should prompt abdominal imaging and investigation for acute pancreatitis.

Diagnosis

- Usually based on the history (dietary indiscretion, foreign body ingestion), clinical findings, and response to symptomatic treatment.
- Complete blood count and chemistry profile are not necessary unless there are systemic signs (fever, abdominal pain).
- Fecal flotation, *Giardia* ELISA.

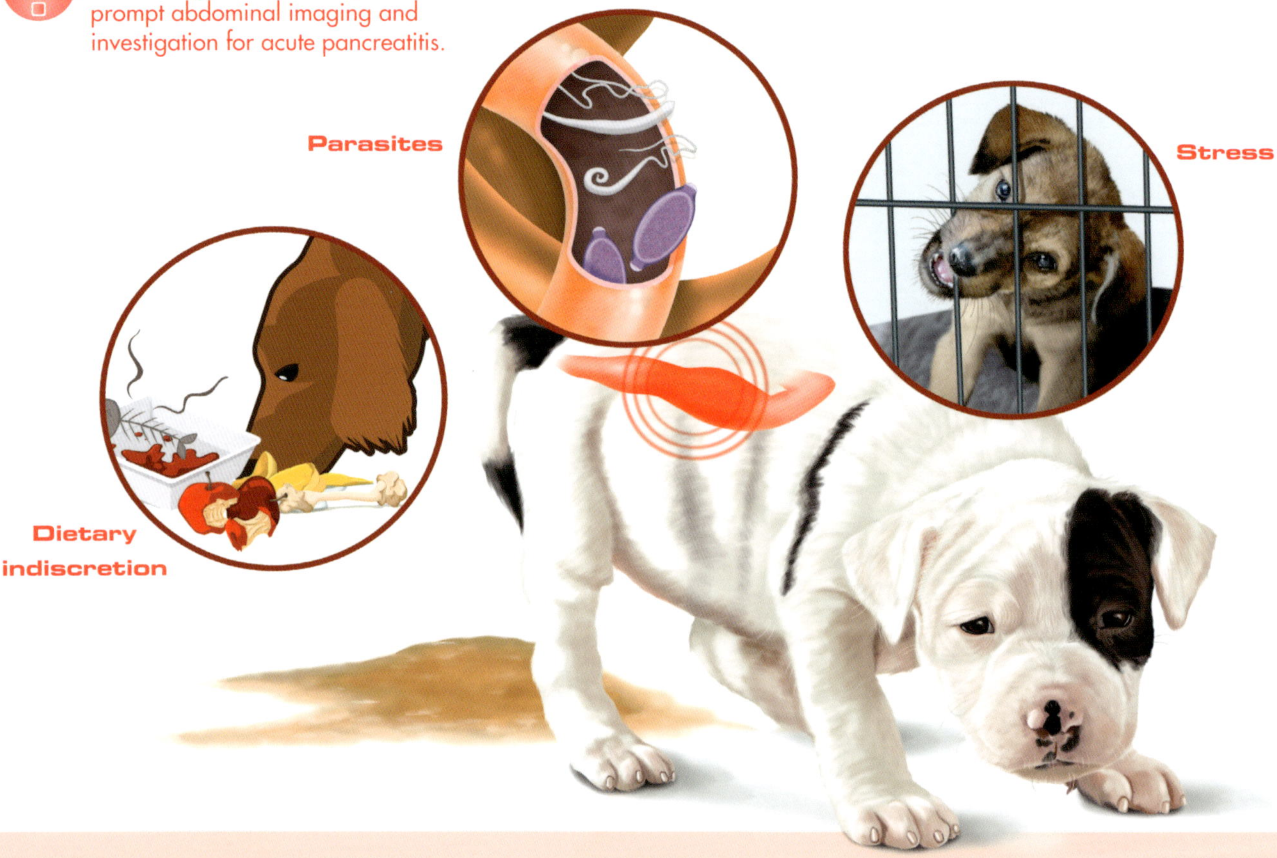

Treatment

- Small, frequent amounts of a highly digestible, low-residue (boiled chicken and rice or a commercial gastrointestinal diet) or fiber-enriched diet.
- Probiotics to decrease the duration of acute diarrhea.
- Empirical deworming (fenbendazole).
- Fluid therapy in case of dehydration.

Prognosis

- Good to excellent for complete recovery in uncomplicated cases of acute colitis.

Most cases of acute colitis are self-resolving and do not require antibiotics such as metronidazole.

DISEASES OF THE LARGE INTESTINE

27 Infectious colitis

Protozoal infection
Tritrichomonas blagburni (formerly *T. foetus*)

- Young cats with a history of dense housing (cattery, shelter).
- Waxing and waning large bowel diarrhea ± hematochezia.
- **Diagnosis:** direct fecal saline smear or PCR.
- **Treatment:** ronidazole once daily. Increased risk of neurotoxicosis with twice-daily dosing.
- **Prognosis:** generally good, although persistent infection may occur.

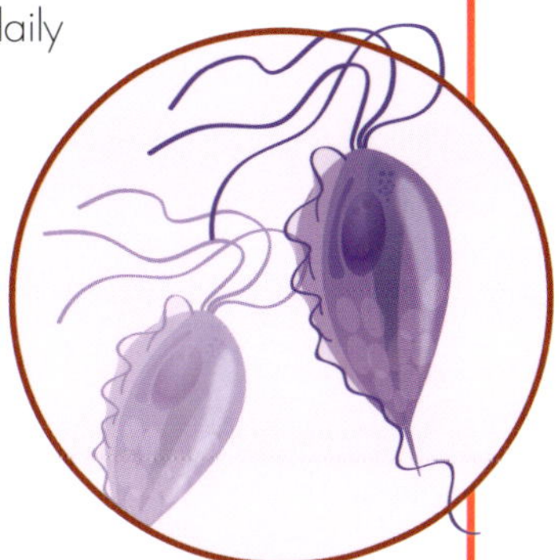

Fungal infection
Pythiosis (*Pythium insidiosum*)

- Young, large-breed dogs exposed to warm freshwater habitats. Uncommon in cats.
- Severe segmental transmural thickening, most often in the pylorus, duodenum, and ileocolic junction.
- Weight loss, vomiting, regurgitation, diarrhea, hematochezia, signs of partial bowel obstruction.
- **Diagnosis:** cytology or biopsy to visualize fungal hyphae. ELISA to detect serum antibodies.
- **Treatment:** aggressive surgical resection, postsurgical antifungal therapy.
- **Prognosis:** guarded to grave when complete excision is not possible.

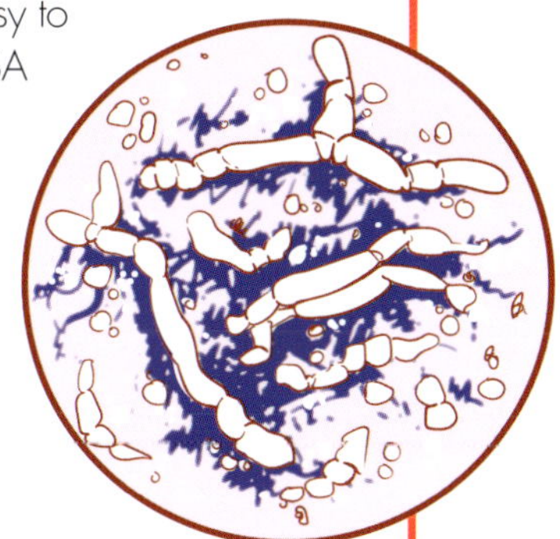

Algal infection
Prototheca

- Young dogs. Uncommon in cats.
- Granulomatous or pyogranulomatous inflammation.
- Intermittent bloody large bowel diarrhea.
- Systemic dissemination (kidney, liver, heart, brain, eye) may occur.
- **Diagnosis:** cytology or biopsy to visualize the organisms.
- **Treatment:** aggressive treatment with amphotericin B and itraconazole, with or without terbinafine.
- **Prognosis:** guarded to grave. The disease is almost always fatal.

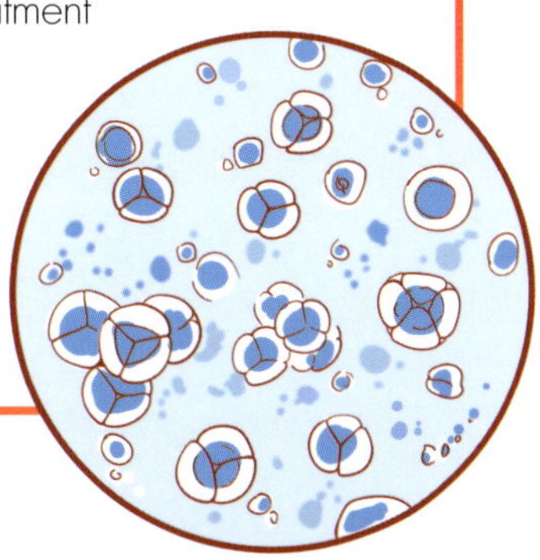

Bacterial infection
Enteropathogens

- *Campylobacter jejuni*, *Clostridioides difficile*, *Clostridium perfringens*, *Salmonella*, *Escherichia coli*.
- Relatively uncommon cause of diarrhea in dogs and cats.
- **Diagnosis:** PCR, ELISA, culture. Use caution, as many of these "pathogens" can be found in healthy animals.
- **Treatment:** supportive care. Antibiotics only when necessary (fever, systemic signs).
- **Prognosis:** generally good.

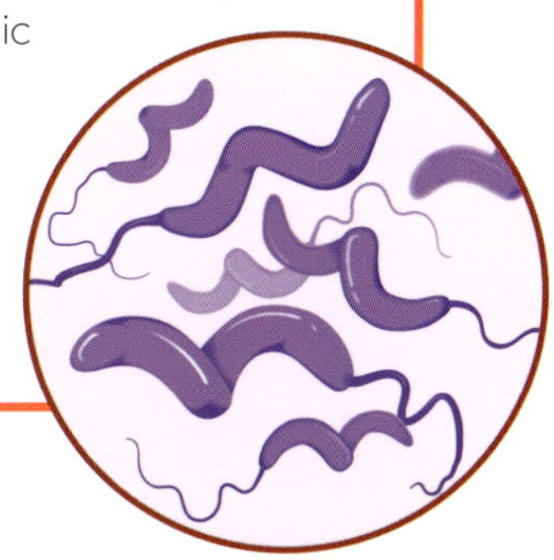

DISEASES OF THE LARGE INTESTINE

28 Idiopathic chronic colitis

Idiopathic chronic inflammatory colitis is diagnosed in animals with chronic (duration >3 weeks) large bowel diarrhea for which no cause can be identified. This involves ruling out systemic (acute pancreatitis) and infectious causes and confirming inflammation on colonic biopsy. Although stress can result in chronic intermittent colitis, it is a disorder of motility and does not result in inflammatory changes on biopsy.

Clinical signs

- Large bowel diarrhea with mucus.
- Vomiting and weight loss if the small intestine is involved.
- Failure to respond to symptomatic treatment.

Diagnosis

- Parallel to that for chronic enteropathy (see Sheet 23).
- Abdominal ultrasound to screen for masses and polyps.
- Colonoscopy to collect biopsy samples and look for polyps. Biopsy may reveal:
  - Lymphoplasmacytic ± eosinophilic colitis: most common.
  - Granulomatous colitis (see Sheet 29).
  - Neutrophilic colitis: suspect bacterial cause.

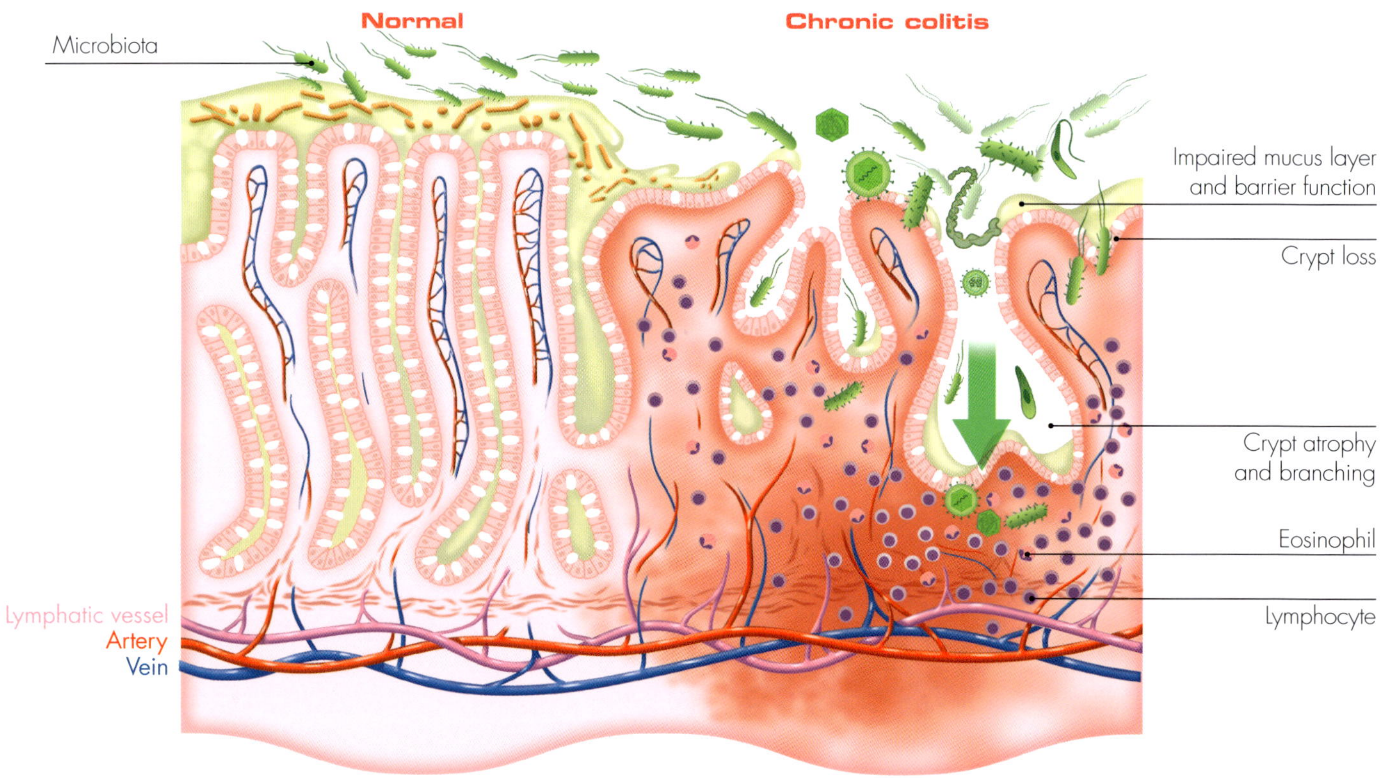

Treatment

- Empirical deworming to rule out parasitic disease.
- Diet trials: fed exclusively (no treats, flavored medications, or oral preventatives) for 2–3 weeks.
  - Easily digestible low-residue diet with fiber, or fiber-enriched diet.
  - Novel protein, limited ingredient, or hydrolyzed diets if there is no response to easily digestible or fiber-enriched diets.
- Probiotic and antibiotic (tylosin, metronidazole) trials.
- Corticosteroids may be indicated for the treatment of idiopathic IBD.

Prognosis

- Variable and largely dependent on the underlying cause.

Endoscopy should be performed prior to antibiotic trials in French Bulldogs and Boxers with large bowel diarrhea (see Sheet 29).

DISEASES OF THE LARGE INTESTINE

29 Granulomatous colitis

Granulomatous colitis, also known as histiocytic ulcerative colitis or Boxer colitis, is caused by invasive *Escherichia coli*. It occurs more frequently in young Boxers, Bulldogs, and French Bulldogs.

Clinical signs

- Onset of disease: often before 2 years of age.
- Large bowel diarrhea (increased frequency, tenesmus, mucus).
- Often hematochezia.
- Weight loss (when ileum also involved).

Diagnosis

- As described for chronic colitis (see Sheet 28).
- Colonoscopy reveals an irregular mucosa with discolored swollen areas interspersed with fistulae and spontaneous bleeding.
- Histopathology shows periodic acid–Schiff (PAS)-positive macrophages in the lamina propria and submucosa.
- Fluorescence in-situ hybridization (FISH) to identify coccobacilli within the colonic mucosa.
- Bacterial culture and sensitivity testing of colonic biopsy samples.

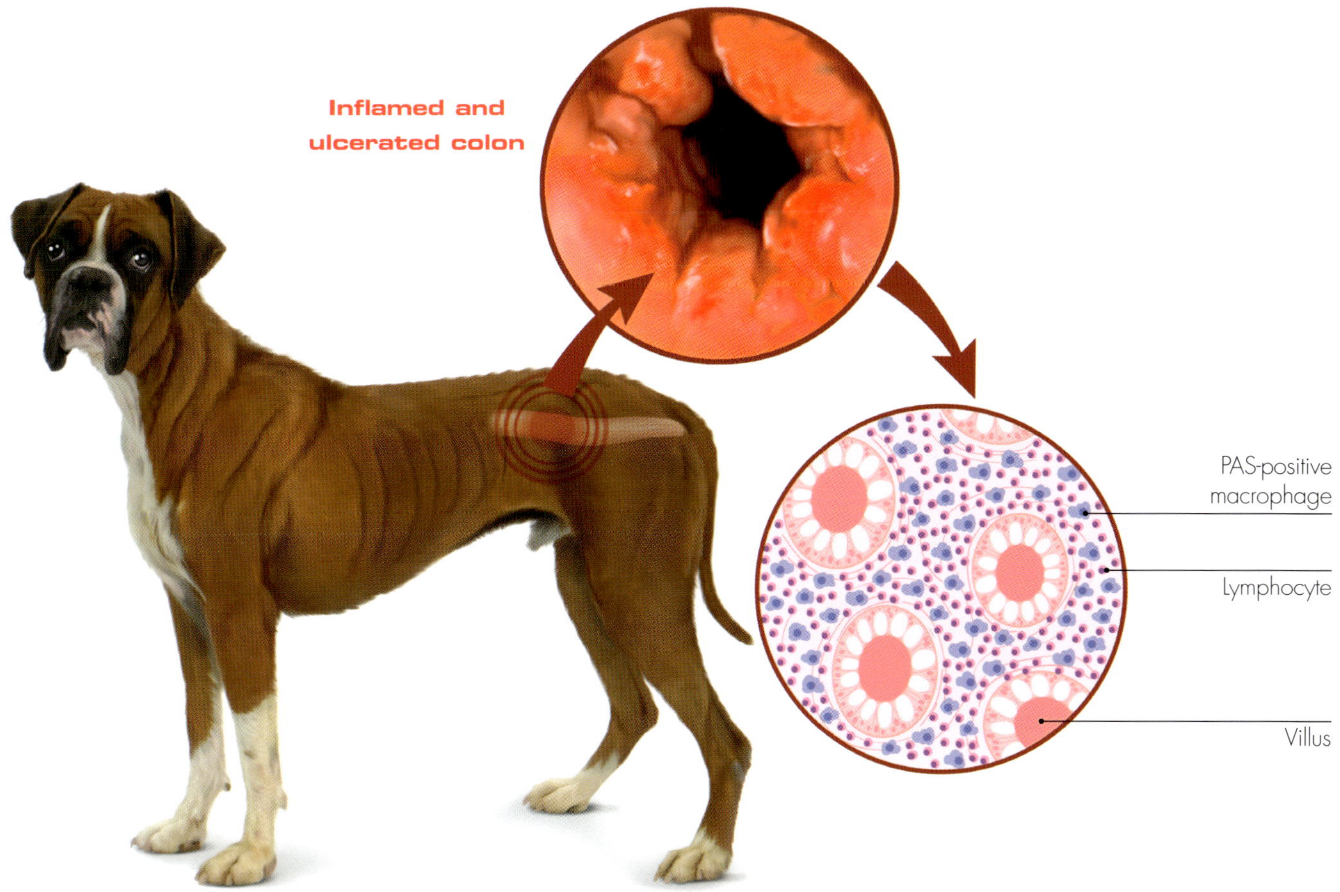

Treatment

- Administration of a fluoroquinolone (enrofloxacin) for 8 weeks typically results in a rapid response. Early discontinuation or poor compliance can create resistant *E. coli*.
- Antimicrobial susceptibility profiling is recommended, as fluroquinolone resistance is widespread.

Prognosis

- Good.
- Failure to administer the full 8-week fluoroquinolone course or a history of previous antibiotic therapy may compromise the prognosis.

DISEASES OF THE LARGE INTESTINE

30 Feline constipation and megacolon

Constipation, obstipation, and megacolon may be observed in cats of any age, sex, or breed but are more common in middle-aged male cats. Constipation may result from inflammation (inflammatory bowel disease), neuromuscular disease (sacral spinal deformity in Manx cats, dysautonomia), endocrine disease (hypothyroidism), metabolic disease (hypokalemia, hypocalcemia, dehydration from chronic kidney disease), medications (opioids, diuretics), environmental changes (inactivity, hospitalization), or mechanical obstruction (foreign material, cancer, pelvic fractures, prostatic disease). The etiopathogenesis of megacolon is not completely understood, but affected cats have permanent loss of colonic structure and function.

Clinical signs

- Reduced, absent, or painful defecation.
- Unproductive attempts to defecate.
- Abdominal pain.
- Vomiting.

Diagnosis

- Complete blood count, chemistry profile, and urinalysis to screen for metabolic causes.
- Abdominal radiographs to characterize the severity of impaction and identify predisposing factors.
- Abdominal ultrasound.
- Colonoscopy and colonic biopsy.

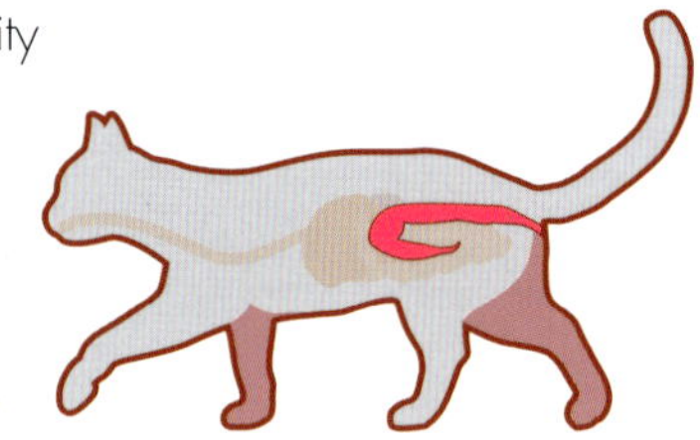

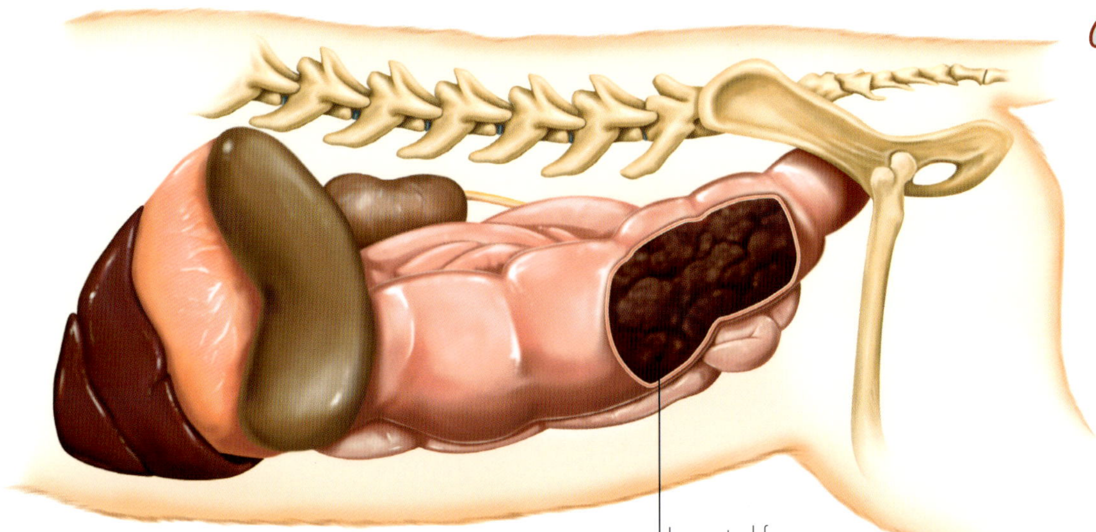

Treatment

- Initial mild episodes can be managed on an outpatient basis:
  - Fiber-enriched diet for constipation and low-residue diet for megacolon.
  - Oral laxatives: lactulose, polyethylene glycol.
  - Colonic prokinetic agents: cisapride.
  - Water enemas.
  - Probiotics can help cats with constipation ± megacolon.
- Manual extraction of impacted feces when colonic impaction is severe.
- Subtotal colectomy may be necessary in cats with idiopathic dilated megacolon.

Prognosis

- Cats with mild to moderate constipation generally respond to medical management.
- Cats refractory to medical management that develop obstipation and dilated megacolon eventually require a colectomy. The prognosis is fair if surgery is possible.

DISEASES OF THE RECTUM AND ANUS

31 Anal sac impaction and infection

The most common cause of inflammation or infection of the anal sacs is ductal obstruction that prevents normal secretion. As a result, proliferation of bacteria and secondary infections occur.

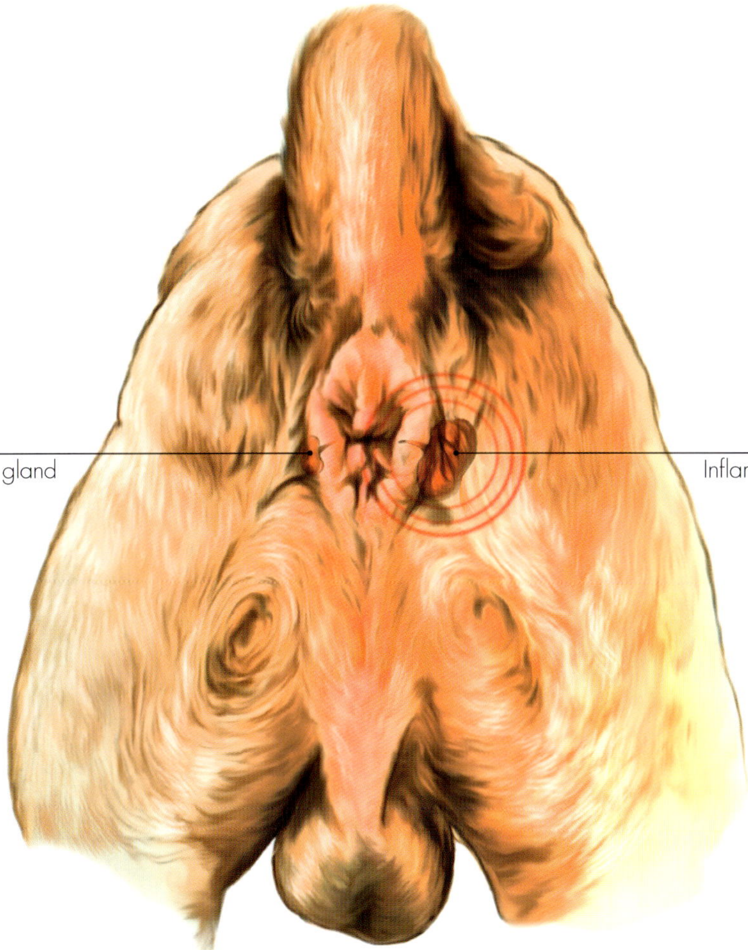

Clinical signs

- Anal pruritus resulting in "tail chasing" behavior and scooting.
- In severe cases, pain may result in dyschezia, tenesmus, reluctance to defecate, and reluctance to sit.

Diagnosis

- Palpable or visual evidence of perianal swelling at the 4 o'clock or 8 o'clock positions lateral to the anus.
- Digital rectal examination (under sedation) to confirm the presence of enlarged and painful anal sacs.
- Expression of purulent or bloody material:
  - Cytology to detect intracellular bacteria (infection).
  - Culture.

Treatment

- Manual emptying and flushing with warm saline or antiseptic solutions (chlorhexidine).
- Abscessed anal sacs must be surgically opened and flushed under general anesthesia every 3–4 days.
- Broad-spectrum oral antibiotics (amoxicillin–clavulanate, cephalexin) for 10–14 days in severe, resistant, or recurrent cases.
- Warm compress to reduce swelling and pain.
- Continued regular gentle expression of anal sacs to prevent recurrence.
- Diet modification: fiber-enriched ± hydrolyzed or limited ingredient diet.
- Anal sacculectomy for recurrent anal sacculitis unresponsive to medical management.

Prognosis

- Most cases respond to medical management.
- Anal sacculectomy may be necessary.

DISEASES OF THE RECTUM AND ANUS

32 Perianal fistula

Perianal fistula, or anal furunculosis, is a chronic, progressive inflammatory disease in dogs characterized by one or more ulcerated fistulas or draining tracts affecting the perianal skin and associated tissues. Perianal fistulas most commonly affect middle-aged to older large-breed dogs with a broad-based tail and low tail carriage. German Shepherd Dogs and their mixes are particularly predisposed, but other breeds can also be affected. The cause remains unknown, but an immune-mediated mechanism in genetically susceptible dogs is suspected. Food allergies may also play a role in some dogs.

Clinical signs

- Perineal licking, self-mutilation.
- Dyschezia, tenesmus.
- Hematochezia.
- Purulent perianal discharge.
- Fecal incontinence in advanced cases due to scaring and anal stenosis or damage to the sphincter muscles and nerves.

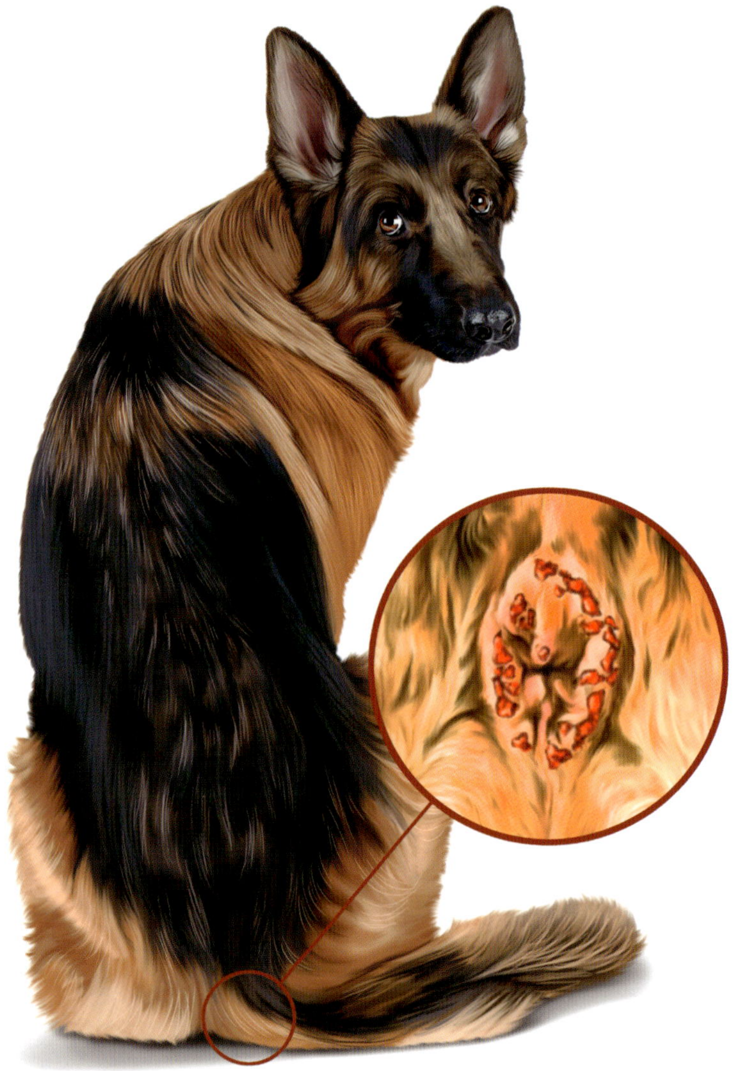

50% of dogs with perianal fistulas have concurrent colitis.

Diagnosis

- Based on signalment, history, clinical findings, and rectal examination under sedation or anesthesia.
- Exclusion of other disorders: anal sac impaction or infection, perianal tumors (adenocarcinomas), untreated bite wounds.

Treatment

- Cyclosporine weaned to the lowest effective dose or transitioned to topical tacrolimus.
- Hypoallergenic diet (hydrolyzed or novel protein).
- Laxatives to lessen pain during defecation.
- Keeping the perianal area clipped, clean, and dry to decrease perianal bacterial populations.
- Surgery has a high complication rate and is only recommended when intensive medical treatment fails.

Prognosis

- Most cases achieve complete remission, but long-term immunosuppressive therapy may be necessary.

DISEASES OF THE RECTUM AND ANUS

33 Apocrine gland anal sac adenocarcinoma (AGASACA)

AGASACA is a rare tumor arising from the anal sacs that occurs less frequently than benign adenomas. Typically, it only affects one anal sac, but bilateral tumors can occur. AGASACA can be very aggressive, with high metastatic rates (50%–80%) at the time of diagnosis. The most common sites of metastasis are the sublumbar lymph nodes, followed by the lungs and the lumbar/pelvic bones.

Clinical signs

- Hematochezia.
- Tenesmus.
- Dyschezia.
- Flattened stools.
- Perianal swelling.
- Signs of hypercalcemia (e.g., increased urination).

Diagnosis

- Mass palpated on rectal examination.
- Cytology and/or histopathology.
- Hypercalcemia may be present (27%).
- Given the high rate of metastasis, staging should include thoracic radiographs and abdominal ultrasound.

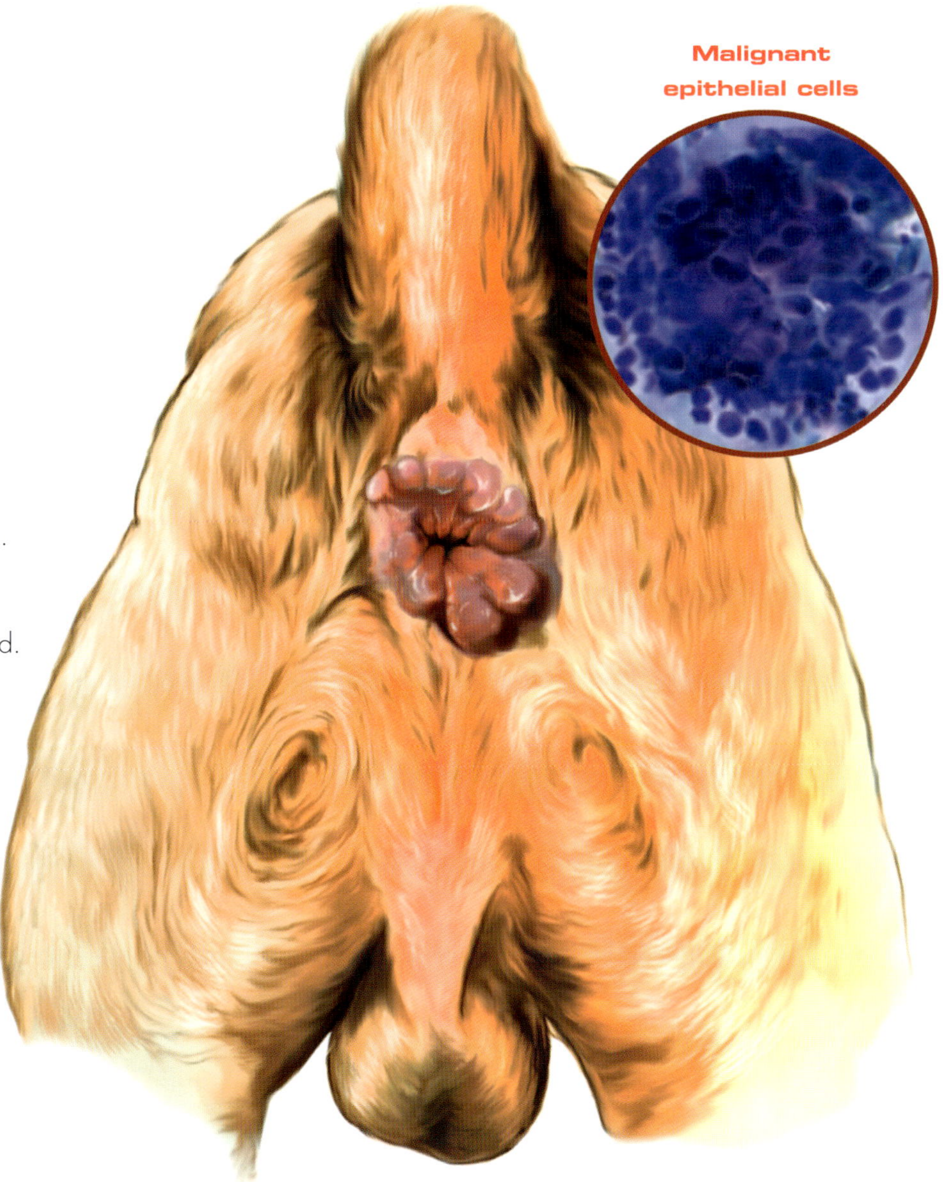

Treatment

- Surgical resection of the primary tumor and enlarged metastatic sublumbar lymph nodes.
- Adjuvant chemotherapy and/or radiation therapy may be considered.

Prognosis

- Surgical resection, either alone or in combination with chemotherapy and/or radiation, leads to a median survival time of 16–18 months.

MISCELLANEOUS GASTROINTESTINAL DISEASES

34 Gastrointestinal foreign bodies

A gastrointestinal foreign body (FB) is any ingested extraneous item (e.g., strings, toys, leashes, clothing, sticks, bones). The resulting clinical signs and complications are associated with the location, duration, and degree of obstruction, as well as with the type of FB material. For example, long-standing FBs can result in tissue necrosis with or without bacterial septicemia, whereas heavy metal–containing FBs can cause toxicity. FBs may be found incidentally during imaging, pass on their own, result in transient signs of gastroenteritis, or cause life-threatening obstruction.

Clinical signs

- Esophageal FBs: dysphagia, regurgitation, gagging, hypersalivation.
- Gastric FBs: intermittent or frequent vomiting, poor appetite, abdominal pain, hypochloremic metabolic alkalosis.
- Intestinal FBs: vomiting, abdominal pain, anorexia, diarrhea.

Diagnosis

- Radiographs to confirm FBs and document obstructive patterns.
- Barium contrast studies or abdominal ultrasound.

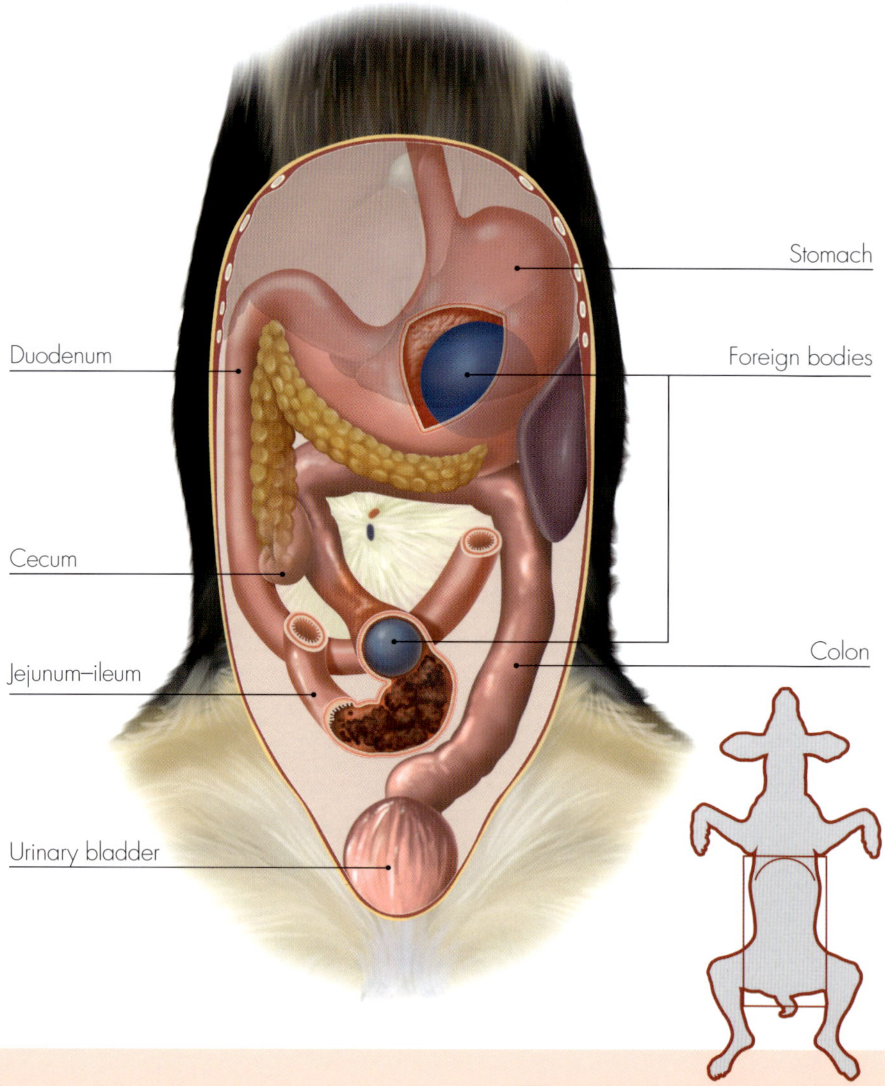

Treatment

- Removal of partially or completely obstructive FBs.
- Esophageal/gastric FBs: endoscopy ± surgery.
  - Distal esophageal FBs may be pushed into the stomach to be digested (bones, food) or removed via gastrotomy.
  - Esophagostomy may be necessary but should be avoided if possible.
  - Friable or numerous gastric FBs (grass, hair): gastrotomy.
- Intestinal FBs: surgery (gastrotomy or enterotomy ± resection of damaged tissue).
- Colonic FBs: colonoscopy ± surgery.

Prognosis

- Good in uncomplicated cases.
- Increased mortality in patients with longer duration of clinical signs, linear FBs, perforation, peritonitis, sepsis, or several enterotomies.

MISCELLANEOUS GASTROINTESTINAL DISEASES

35 Intussusception

Gastrointestinal intussusceptions are an uncommon form of bowel obstruction that occur when a migrating peristaltic wave reaches a fixed or noncontractile segment. Usually, a proximal segment of the gastrointestinal tract (intussusceptum) telescopes into the lumen of the adjacent distal segment (intussuscipiens). The most common sites are the jejunum and the ileocolic junction. Intussusceptions occur most often in young animals (<1 year) but may be seen in older animals secondary to intestinal cancer. Most intussusceptions in dogs are idiopathic; however, any disturbance of intestinal motility (e.g., viral enteritis, cancer, foreign bodies, prior abdominal surgery) may lead to intussusception.

Intussusceptions can be chronic or intermittent (i.e., they reduce themselves spontaneously and then reform).

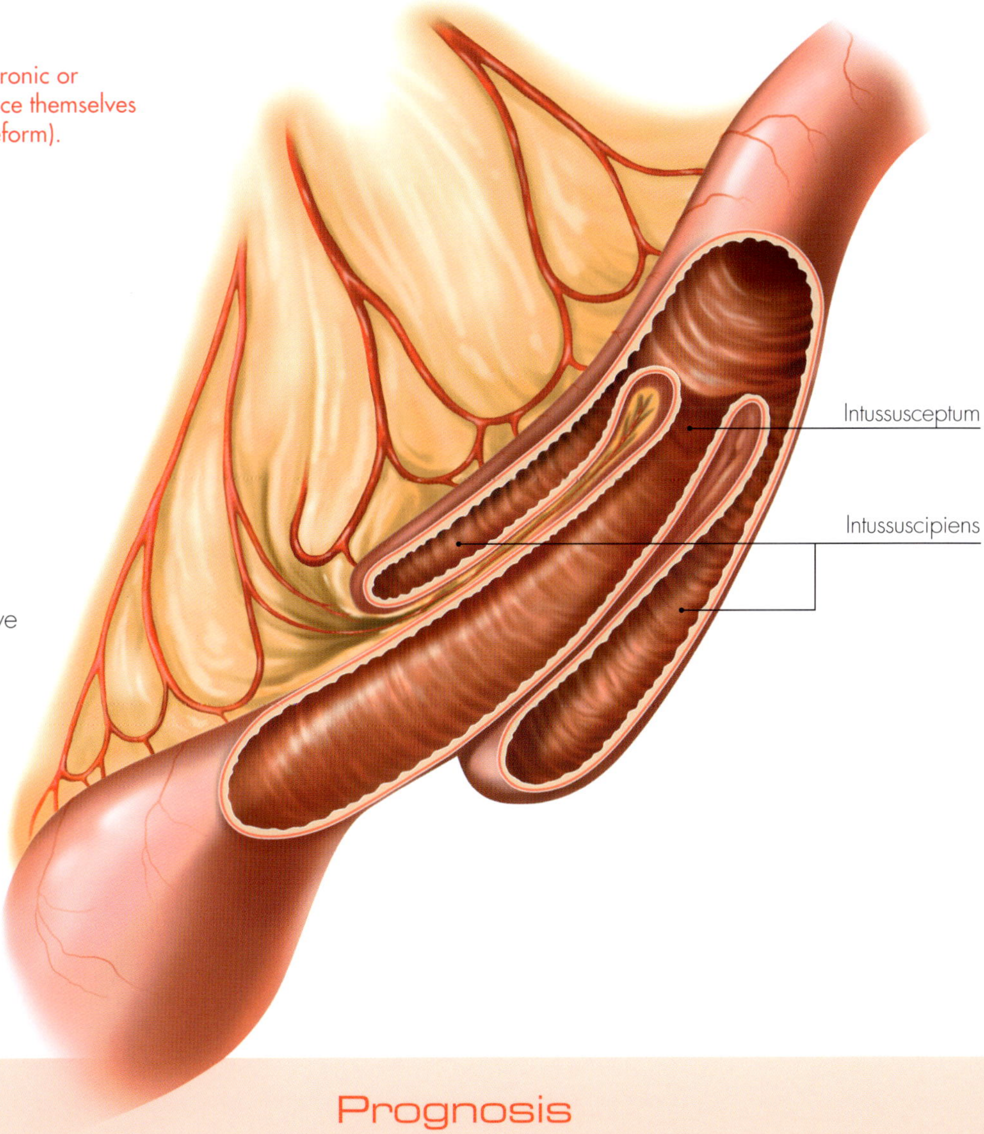

Clinical signs

- Vomiting.
- Diarrhea.
- Abdominal pain.
- Anorexia.

Diagnosis

- The intussusception can often be palpated as an abdominal mass.
- Abdominal radiographs: obstructive pattern if complete obstruction.
- Abdominal ultrasound.

Treatment

- Surgery: manual reduction.
  - Enterectomy and anastomosis if the affected segment is not reducible, not viable, or associated with a mass lesion.
- Percutaneous manual reduction may be successful, but the chance of recurrence is high.
- Some intussusceptions spontaneously resolve with anesthesia.

Prognosis

- Depends on the underlying cause. Good long-term prognosis in idiopathic cases.
- Complications: recurrence, dehiscence of intestinal anastomosis, ileus, intestinal obstruction, peritonitis, short bowel syndrome.
- Recurrence rate in dogs: 11%–27%. Enteroplication can be performed at the time of surgery to prevent recurrence.

MISCELLANEOUS GASTROINTESTINAL DISEASES

36 Gastrointestinal parasites

Gastrointestinal parasites are a common cause of gastrointestinal signs in young dogs and cats.

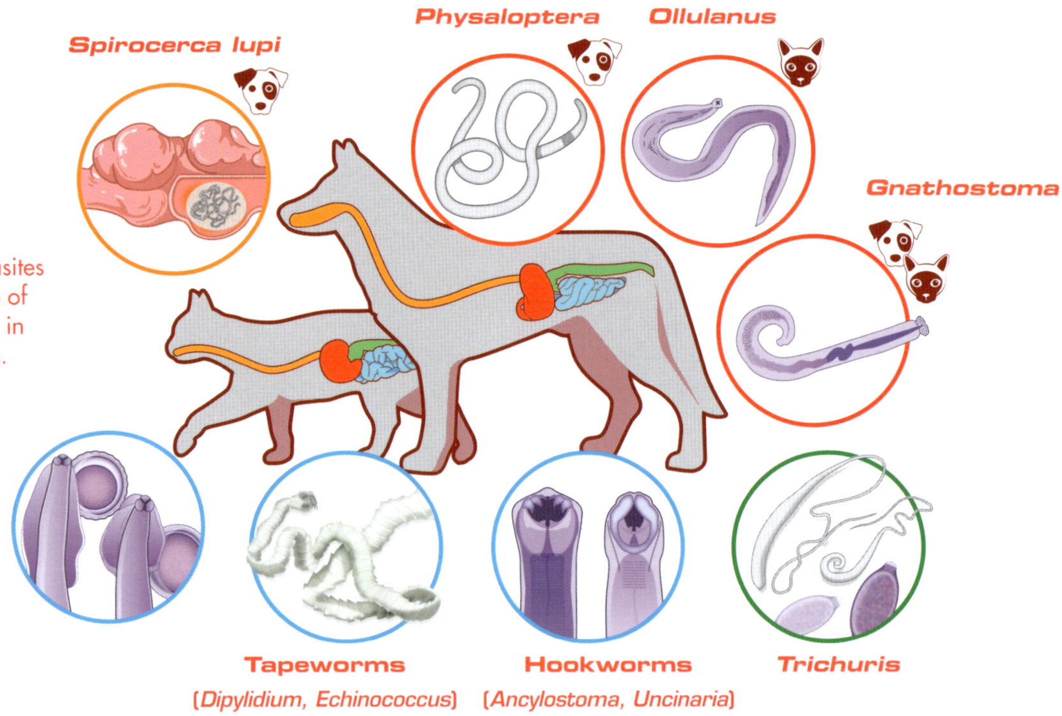

Parasite	Host	Location	Clinical signs	Diagnosis	Treatment
Spirocerca lupi	Dog	Esophagus, stomach	Regurgitation, vomiting, granulomas, esophageal cancer	Endoscopy, fecal flotation, survey radiographs	Avermectins
Physaloptera	Dog	Stomach, small intestine	Chronic vomiting	Identification of adult worms on endoscopy or in vomit Fecal flotation not reliable (low worm burden, clear eggs)	Endoscopic removal Pyrantel pamoate
Ollulanus	Cat	Stomach	Chronic vomiting, weight loss, anorexia	Identification of adult worms in vomit or gastric lavage fluid	Tetramisole, fenbendazole+oxfendazole
Gnathostoma	Dog, cat	Stomach, systemic migration	Vomiting, weight loss, anorexia	Fecal flotation with centrifugation	Albendazole, fenbendazole
Roundworms *Toxocara* *Toxascaris* *Baylisascaris*	Dog, cat	Small intestine	Failure to gain weight, poor haircoat, pot-bellied appearance	Fecal flotation with centrifugation	Fenbendazole, milbemycin oxime, moxidectin, pyrantel pamoate
Hookworms *Ancylostoma* *Uncinaria*	Dog, cat	Small intestine	Failure to gain weight, poor haircoat, dehydration, melena, anemia	Fecal flotation with centrifugation	Fenbendazole, milbemycin oxime, moxidectin, pyrantel pamoate Supportive care for severe infections
Tapeworms *Dipylidium* *Echinococcus*	Dog, cat	Small intestine	Rarely pathologic Anal irritation	Visualization of proglottids in perineal area	Flea control Praziquantel
Whipworms *Trichuris*	Dog, cat	Small intestine, large intestine	Often asymptomatic Severe infection: bloody diarrhea, dehydration, anemia	Fecal flotation with centrifugation	Fenbendazole, febantel: repeat in 3 weeks and again in 3 months

MISCELLANEOUS GASTROINTESTINAL DISEASES

37 Gastrointestinal cancer

Although uncommon, gastrointestinal cancers in dogs and cats are aggressive and have poor outcomes despite therapy.

Prevalence

Most common gastrointestinal cancers:

	Dogs	Cats
Stomach	• Adenocarcinoma (80%)	• Lymphoma
Intestine	• Lymphoma • Adenocarcinoma • Leiomyosarcoma • Gastrointestinal stromal tumor	• Lymphoma • Adenocarcinoma • Mast cell tumor

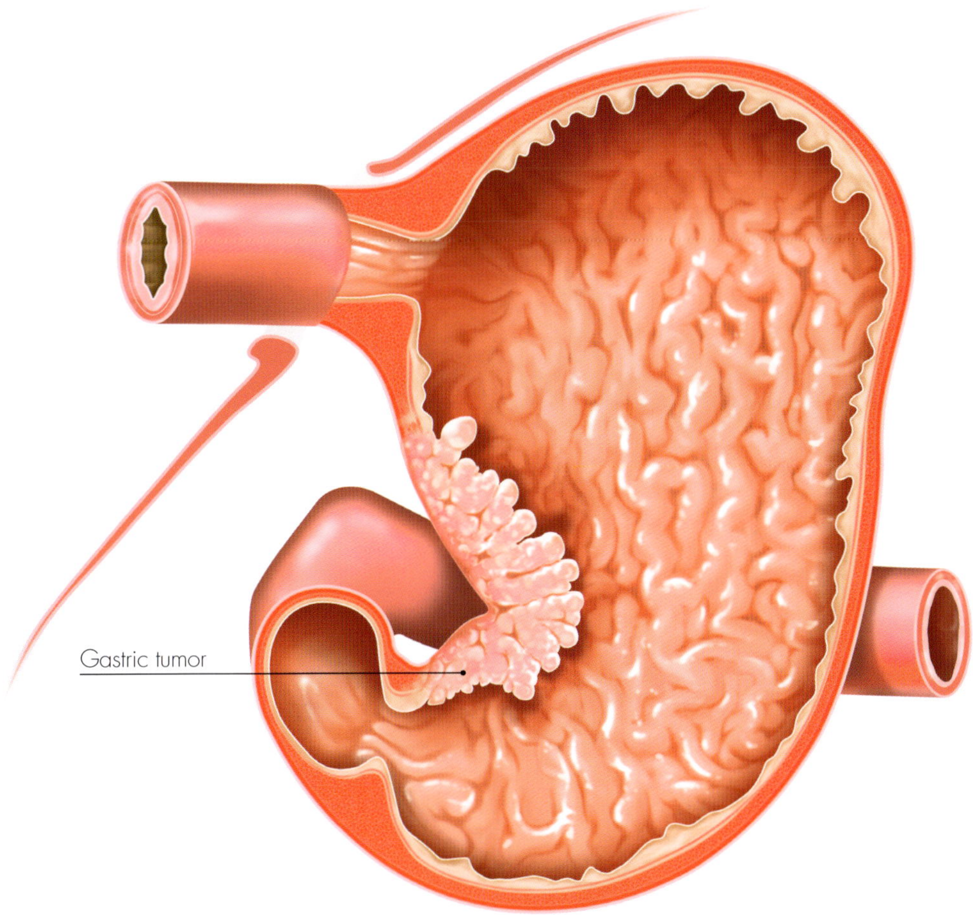

Clinical signs

Dependent on the location.

- Vomiting.
- Weight loss.
- Anorexia.
- Hematemesis, melena, hematochezia.
- Diarrhea.
- Tenesmus, constipation (colonic, rectal).

Diagnosis

- Contrast abdominal radiographs.
- Abdominal ultrasound:
  - Small intestinal wall thickening ± loss of layering and masses.
  - Colonic and gastric masses (normal study does not rule out).
  - Evaluation of local lymph nodes.
  - Fine needle aspiration.
- Endoscopy:
  - Mucosal gastric, duodenal, and colonic masses.
  - Biopsy.
- Surgical biopsy: jejunal masses + lymph nodes.

Treatment

- Surgical resection: gastrointestinal adenocarcinoma, smooth muscle tumor.
- Chemotherapy: lymphoma, evidence of metastatic disease.

Prognosis

- Dependent on the type and location of the tumor and the presence of metastasis.

MISCELLANEOUS GASTROINTESTINAL DISEASES

38 Acute abdomen

Acute abdomen is any condition associated with a sudden onset of severe abdominal pain that often requires surgical intervention. Examples include gastric dilatation and volvulus, septic peritonitis, bile peritonitis, gastrointestinal obstruction (foreign bodies, intussusception), bleeding abdominal masses (splenic, hepatic), pyometra, mesenteric volvulus, organ torsion, urinary tract obstruction, and rupture of the urinary tract. Diseases such as acute pancreatitis, gastrointestinal ulceration, pyelonephritis, and acute hepatitis can result in abdominal pain but do not require surgical intervention.

Clinical signs

- Tachycardia, tachypnea.
- Restlessness, guarding or splinting of the abdomen.
- Arched back.
- Abdominal distension.
- Gastrointestinal signs: vomiting, anorexia, diarrhea, hypersalivation, retching.
- Poor perfusion parameters: prolonged capillary refill time, poor pulse quality.

Diagnosis

- Abdominal ultrasound.
- Abdominocentesis: comparison of paired fluid and blood samples.
  - Hemoabdomen: paired hematocrit and total protein.
  - Uroabdomen: paired creatinine.
  - Septic peritonitis: intracellular bacteria, culture, paired glucose and lactate.
  - Bile peritonitis: paired total bilirubin.
- Abdominal radiographs: torsion, gastric dilatation and volvulus, obstruction, uroabdomen.

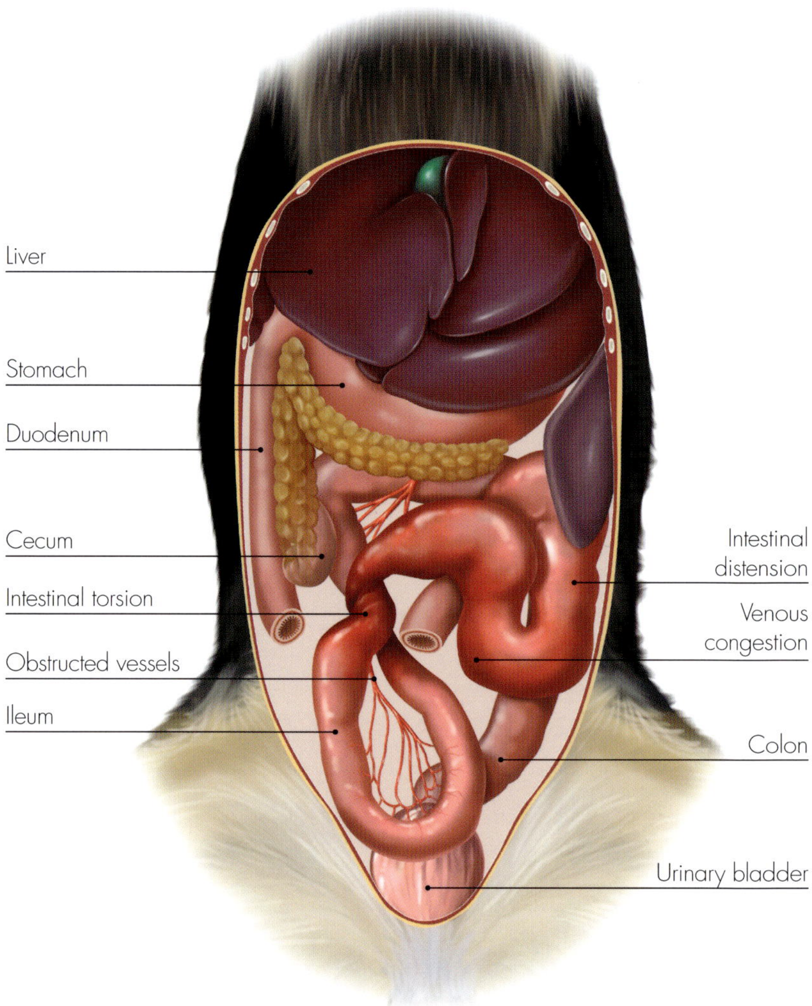

Treatment

- Patient stabilization: intravenous fluids, analgesia, and antibiotics (after culture is taken).
- Surgical intervention to correct the underlying cause.

Prognosis

- Dependent on the underlying cause.
- Good in patients with splenic torsion with early intervention.
- Splenic mass hemoabdomen: hemangiosarcoma (2/3 of cases; poor prognosis), hematoma (1/3 of cases; good prognosis).
- Guarded in patients with septic peritonitis (20%–50% mortality rate).

39 Upper gastrointestinal endoscopy

Esophagus

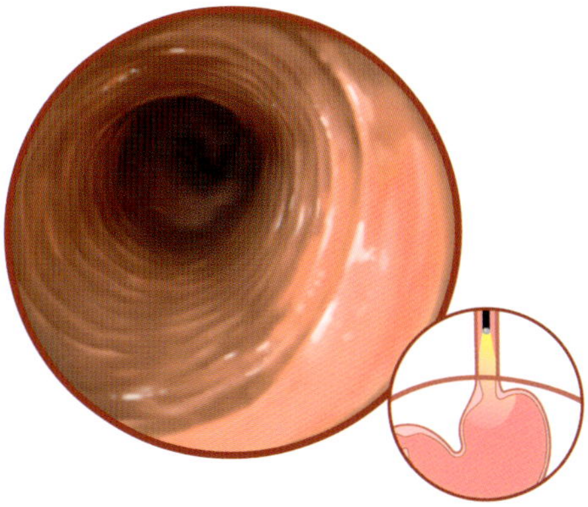

Indications

- Diagnose diseases that disrupt the esophageal, gastric, or duodenal mucosa via visual examination and biopsy.
- Remove esophageal and gastric foreign bodies.

Preparation and patient positioning

- Food is withheld for 12–18 hours before endoscopy. Water should be available up to 2 hours prior to the procedure.
- Left lateral recumbency under anesthesia.

> ! Intubating the pylorus is much easier when insufflation is kept to a minimum. Typically, evaluation of the incisura angularis and cardia is performed after duodenoscopy is finished.

Stomach
(fundus/cardia)

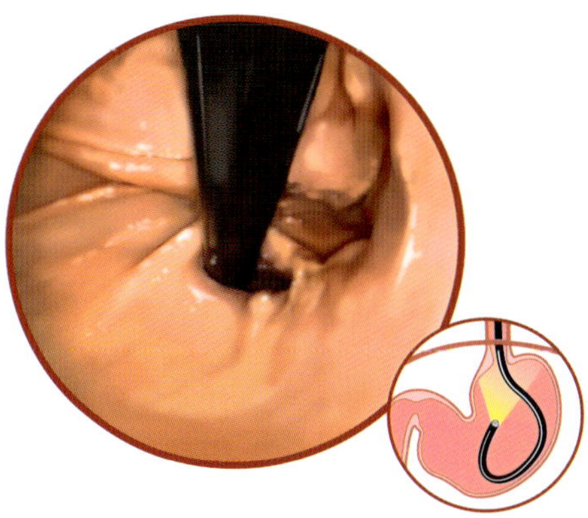

Stomach
(body)

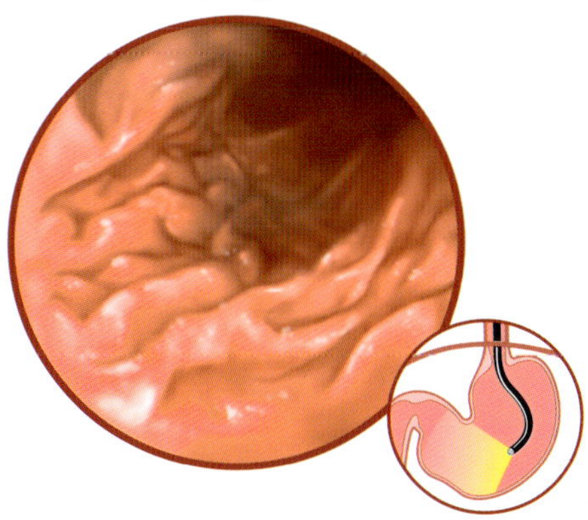

Stomach
(pylorus)

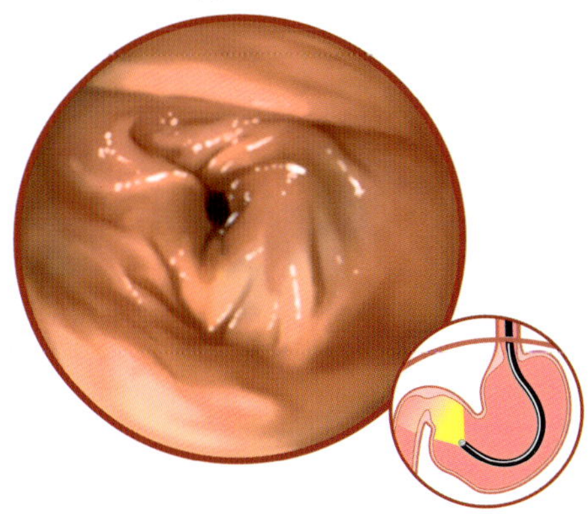

Duodenum
(major duodenal papilla)

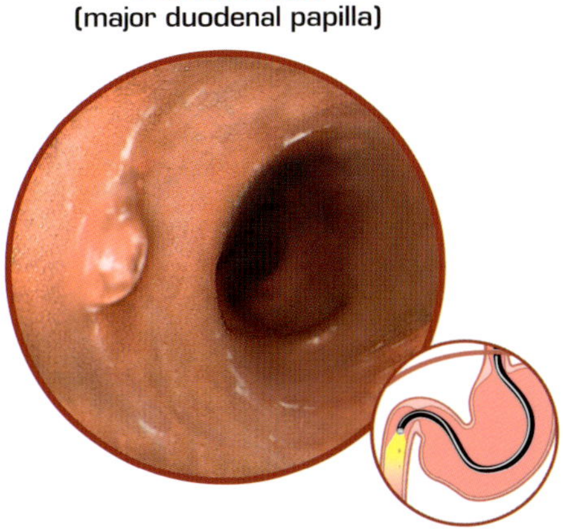

Duodenum
(descending)

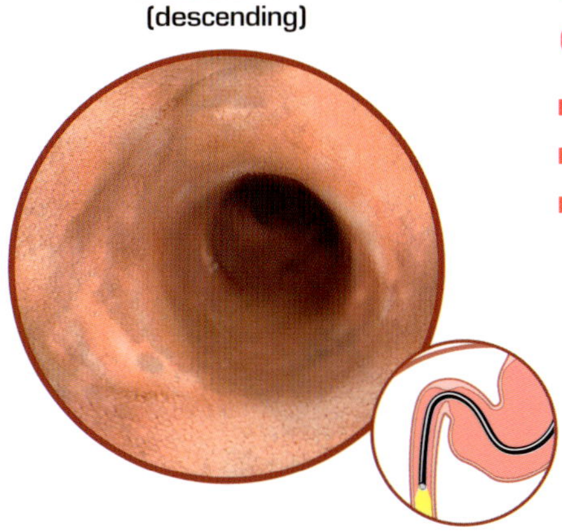

Possible complications

- Gastrointestinal perforation.
- Hemorrhage from blood vessel laceration.
- Anesthetic complications:
  - Aspiration pneumonia.
  - Gastric overdistension that may result in a vasovagal reaction.

40 Ileal intubation and biopsy

Indications

- Diagnose diseases that disrupt the ileal mucosa via visual examination and biopsy.
- Low serum cobalamin (vitamin B_{12}) concentration.
- Protein-losing enteropathy.

Preparation and patient positioning

- Food is withheld for 24–48 hours.
- Polyethylene glycol–containing electrolyte gastrointestinal lavage solution:
  - Administer via nasogastric tube to avoid aspiration and severe complications.
  - 2–3 doses administered 2–4 hours apart the day prior to endoscopy.
  - Premedication with an antiemetic can be considered.
- Warm water enemas.
- Left lateral recumbency under anesthesia.

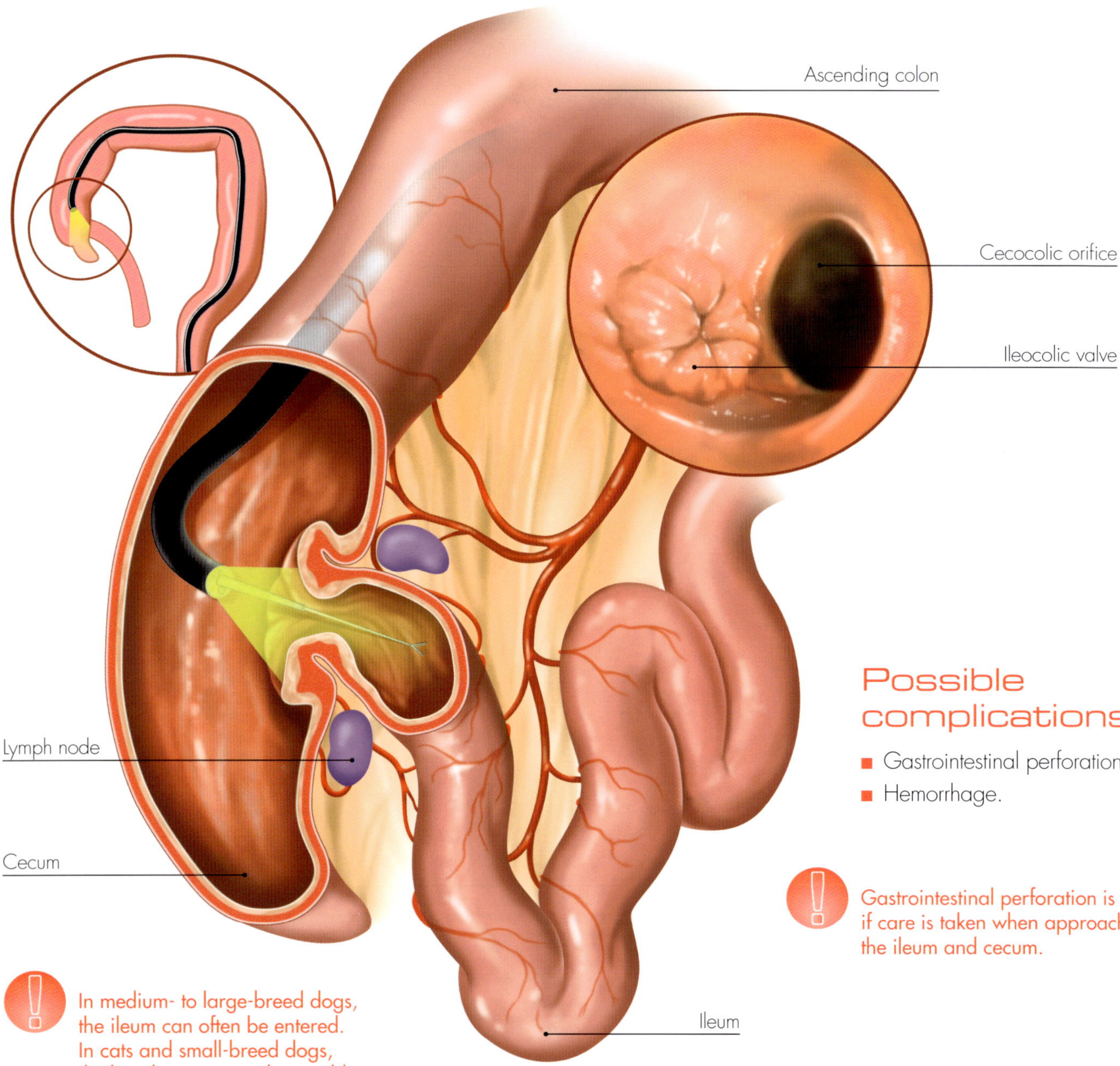

Possible complications

- Gastrointestinal perforation.
- Hemorrhage.

Gastrointestinal perforation is rare if care is taken when approaching the ileum and cecum.

In medium- to large-breed dogs, the ileum can often be entered. In cats and small-breed dogs, ileal intubation is rarely possible.

41 Colonoscopy

Indications

- Diagnose diseases that disrupt the colonic mucosa via visual examination and biopsy.
- Chronic large bowel diarrhea unresponsive to anthelmintics, diet, or fiber.

Colonoscopy allows for evaluation and biopsy of the descending, transverse, and ascending colon. Small polyps and foreign bodies can be removed via colonoscopy.

Preparation and patient positioning

- Food is withheld for 24–48 hours.
- Polyethylene glycol–containing electrolyte gastrointestinal lavage solution:
  - Administer via nasogastric tube to avoid aspiration and severe complications.
  - 2–3 doses administered 2–4 hours apart the day prior to endoscopy.
  - Premedication with an antiemetic can be considered.
- Warm water enemas.
- Left lateral recumbency under anesthesia (right lateral for rigid colonoscopes).

Possible complications

- Gastrointestinal perforation.
- Hemorrhage.

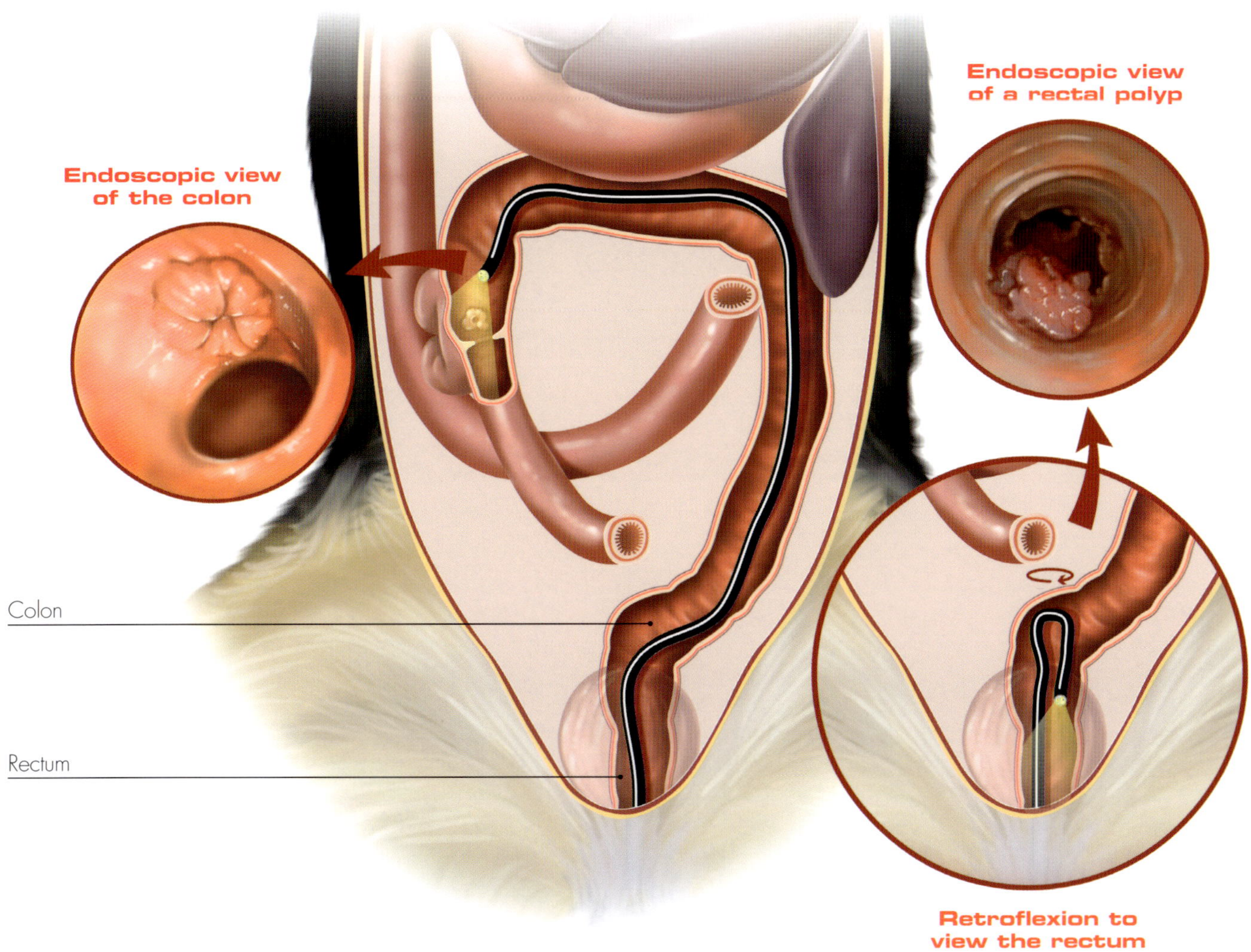

42 Feeding tubes

Feeding tubes are placed to provide nutritional support to patients that have dysorexia (abnormal appetite or change in food-seeking behavior), are critically ill, or have facial or oral trauma that prevents them from eating by mouth. Some patients require temporary feeding tubes following surgery of the upper gastrointestinal tract. Feeding tubes also facilitate medication administration and hydration support (e.g., in patients with kidney disease or free water loss).

! Feeding tubes do not interfere with the ability of the animal to eat or drink by mouth.

Nasoesophageal and nasogastric tubes

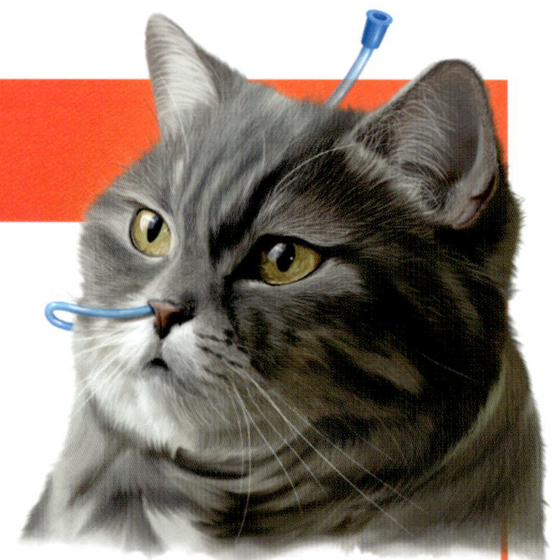

- **Description:** small-diameter tubes that end just before the lower esophageal sphincter (nasoesophageal tubes) or in the stomach (nasogastric tubes).
- **Indications:** short-term (3–7 days) in-hospital enteral nutritional support.
- **Contraindications:**
  - Diseases of the nares, pharynx, larynx, hyoid apparatus, esophagus, or stomach.
  - Thrombocytopenia, platelet dysfunction.

Esophagostomy tubes

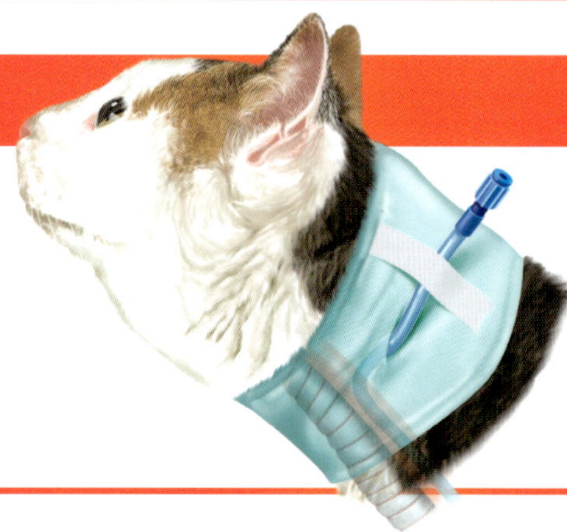

- **Description:** intermediate-diameter tubes that enter on the left side of the neck and end just before the lower esophageal sphincter.
- **Indications:** at-home enteral nutritional support (weeks to years).
  - Hyporexic or anorexic pets.
  - Pets with diseases of the oral or nasal cavity.
- **Contraindications:** primary or secondary esophageal disorders.

Gastrostomy tubes

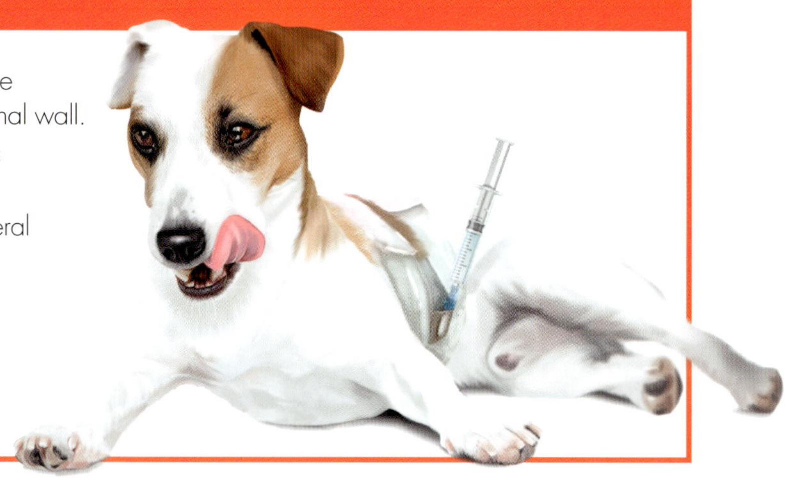

- **Description:** large-diameter tubes that pass directly into the stomach through a small opening in the skin and abdominal wall.
- **Examples:** surgically placed or percutaneous endoscopic gastrostomy (PEG) tubes.
- **Indications:** long-term (months to indefinitely) at-home enteral nutritional support.
  - Pets with diseases of the esophagus or oral cavity.
- **Contraindications:**
  - Diseases of the stomach.
  - Peritonitis, peritoneal effusion.

43 Esophageal balloon dilatation

Indications

- Esophageal strictures.

Procedure

- Fluoroscopy is often utilized to monitor dilatation.
- Under general anesthesia, an endoscope is inserted into the esophagus to visualize the stricture.
- The balloon is inserted through the endoscope and placed in the middle of the stricture.
- The balloon is filled with saline, causing the stricture to break down.
- The process is repeated with progressively larger balloons and/or dilatation pressures.

Possible complications

- Tearing of esophageal lining.
- Formation of diverticula (hollow, pouch-like sacs).
- Esophageal perforation.
- Aspiration pneumonia.

Outcome

- Multiple dilatations are often required.
- Variable success (12%–88%) based on the severity of the stricture.

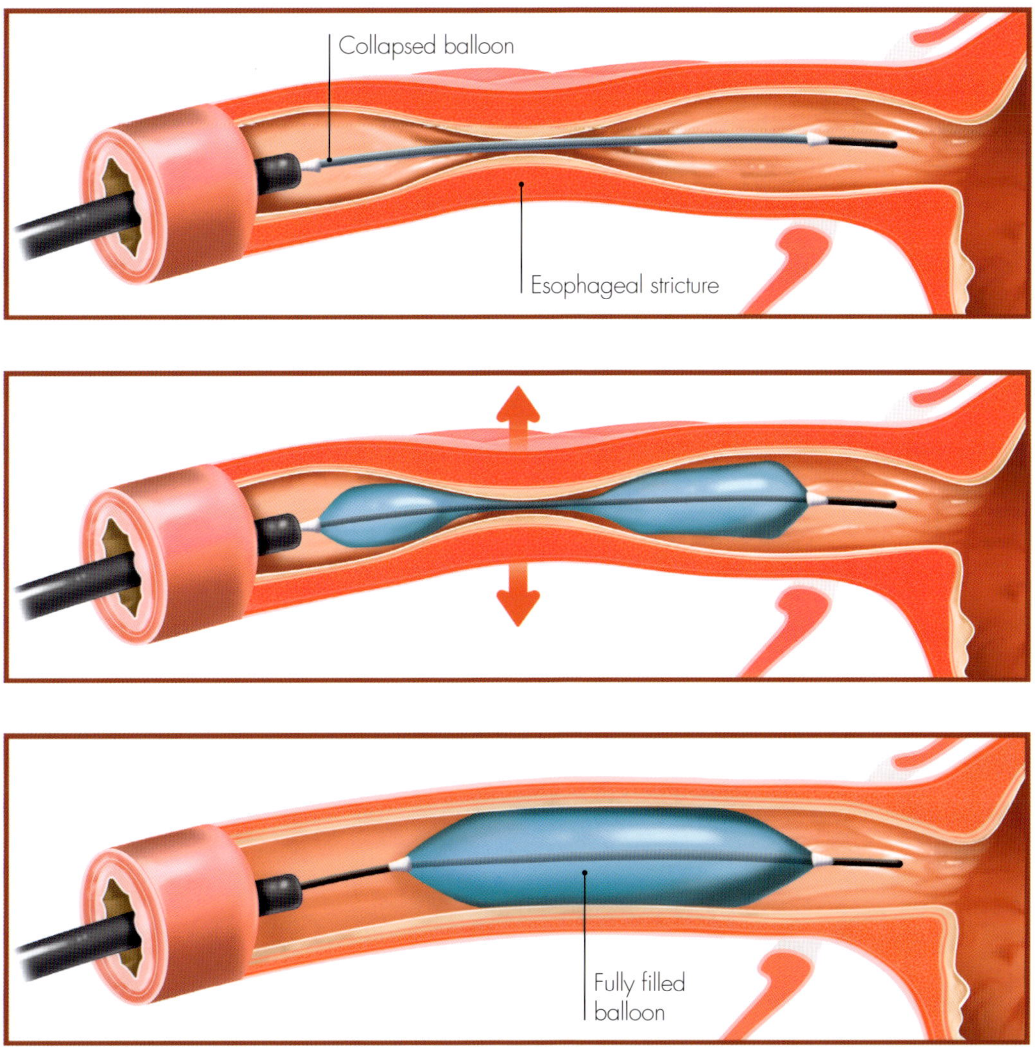

44 Fecal microbiota transplantation (FMT)

FMT is the transfer of intestinal contents from a healthy donor to a diseased recipient with the goal of lessening diarrhea and improving gastrointestinal health.

Indications

- Parvovirus infection.
- Acute or chronic diarrhea.
- Chronic enteropathy unresponsive to diet, deworming, or immunosuppression.

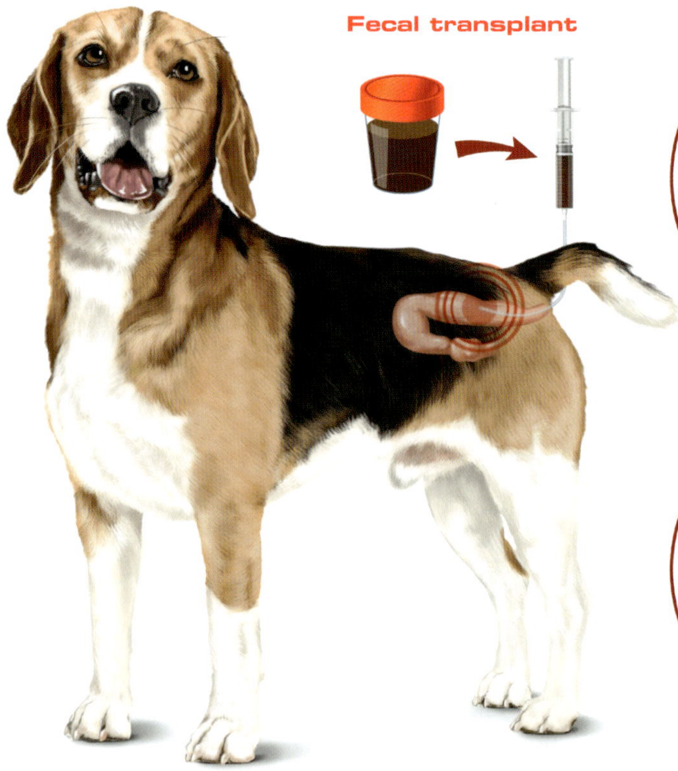

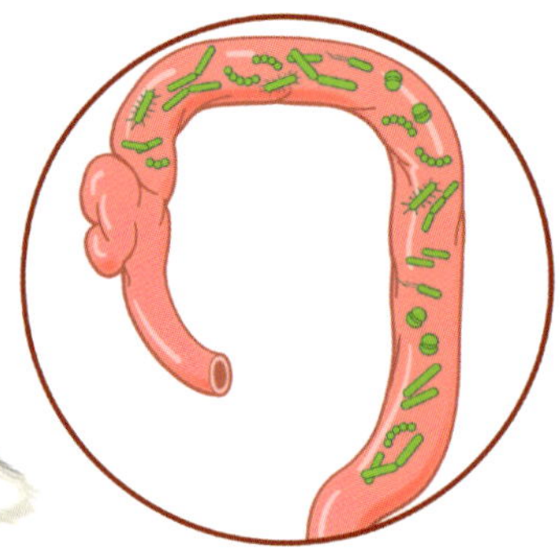

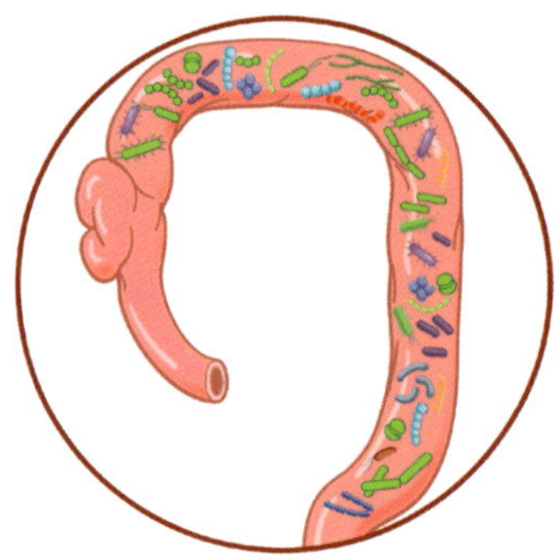

Amount

- 2–6 grams of feces per kilogram of recipient body weight.

Preparation

- Use or freeze feces within 6–12 hours of defecation.
- In a blender, mix one volume of feces with four volumes of 0.9% NaCl until stool is liquefied.
- Filter solid material out using a gauze.

Administration

- 5–10 ml of solution per kilogram of recipient body weight is administered rectally via a large-bore red rubber catheter.
- The recipient should be kept calm for 30 minutes after the procedure. Mild sedation can be helpful.
- Restrict activity and do not feed for 4–6 hours after administration to decrease the chance of defecation.

Donor selection

- No health concerns for the last 6–12 months.
- No history of gastrointestinal disease.
- Normal fecal score.
- Fed a balanced and completely cooked diet.
- Has not received antibiotics in the last 12 months.
- Healthy on physical examination.
- Good body condition score (4–6/9).
- Normal complete blood count and chemistry profile.
- Negative for parasites on fecal flotation.
- Negative *Giardia* ELISA.
- Negative for fecal pathogens (*Salmonella*, *Campylobacter*).
- Fecal dysbiosis index less than 0.

45 Anatomy of the hepatobiliary system

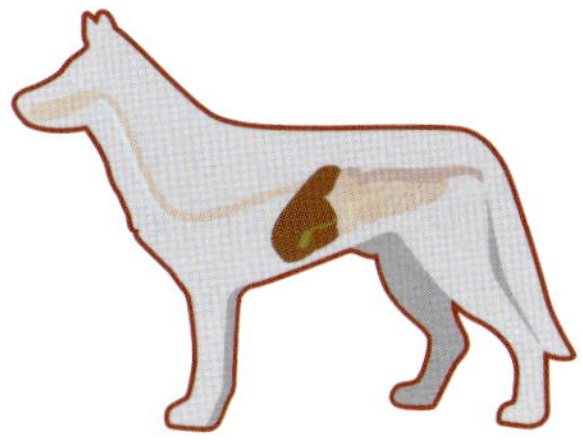

Liver
(visceral surface)

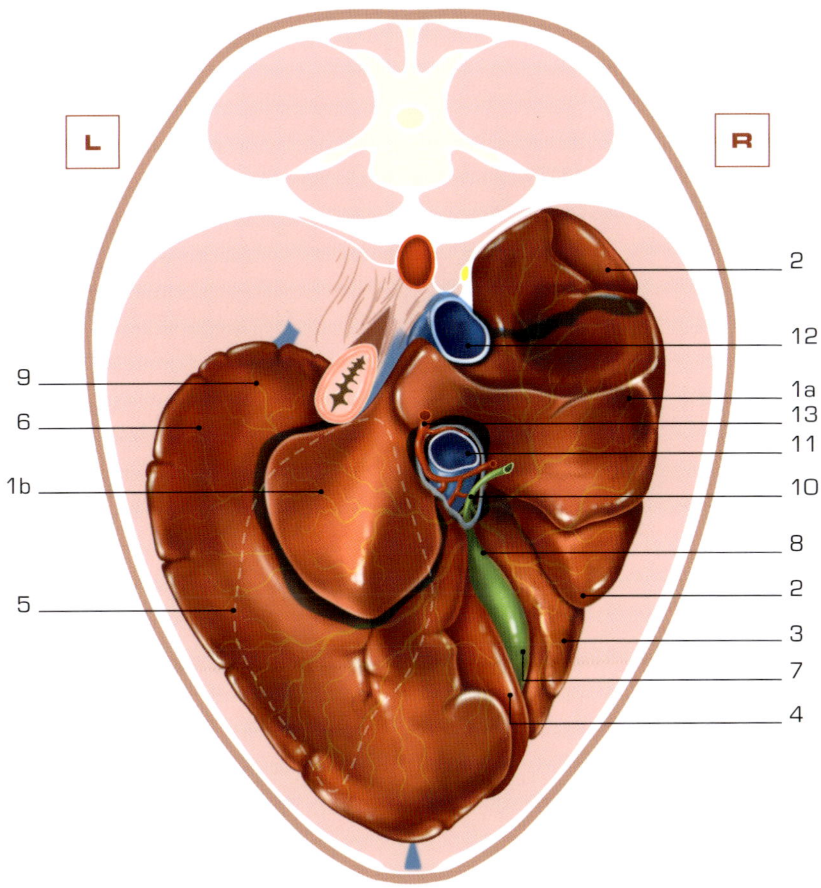

1. Caudate lobe
  1a. Caudate process
  1b. Papillary process
2. Right lateral lobe
3. Right medial lobe
4. Quadrate lobe
5. Left medial lobe
6. Left lateral lobe
7. Gallbladder
8. Cystic duct
9. Hepatic duct
10. Common bile duct
11. Portal vein
12. Caudal vena cava
13. Hepatic artery

Hepatic lobule

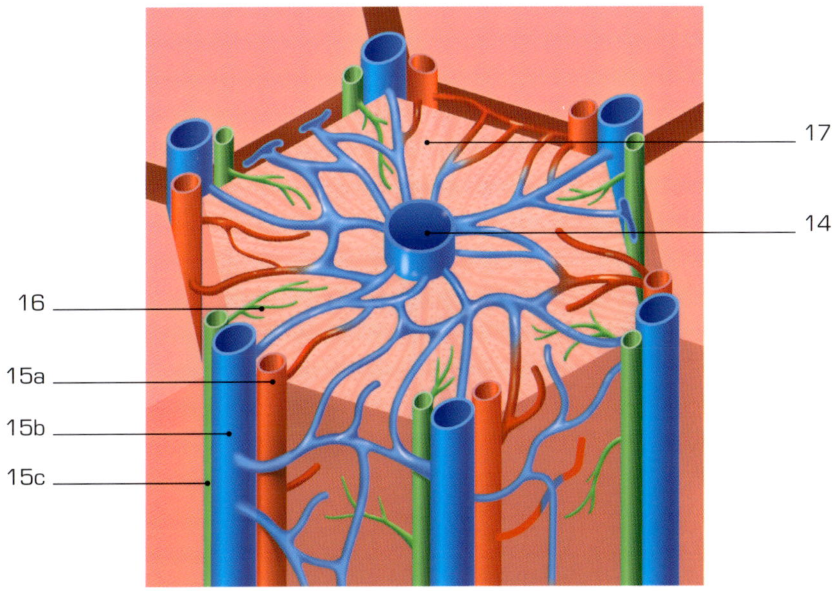

14. Central vein
15. Portal triad
  15a. Hepatic artery
  15b. Portal vein
  15c. Bile duct
16. Bile canaliculus
17. Hepatocytes

46 Regulation of bile secretion

Measuring bile acids (BAs) in the blood before (fasting BAs) and 2 hours after a meal (postprandial BAs) allows for assessment of liver function. If liver function is compromised, fewer BAs are taken out of the blood by the liver. As a result, postprandial BAs are higher in cats and dogs with congenital portosystemic shunts and other causes of decreased liver function. Cholestasis (decreased bile flow) can also result in increased BAs.

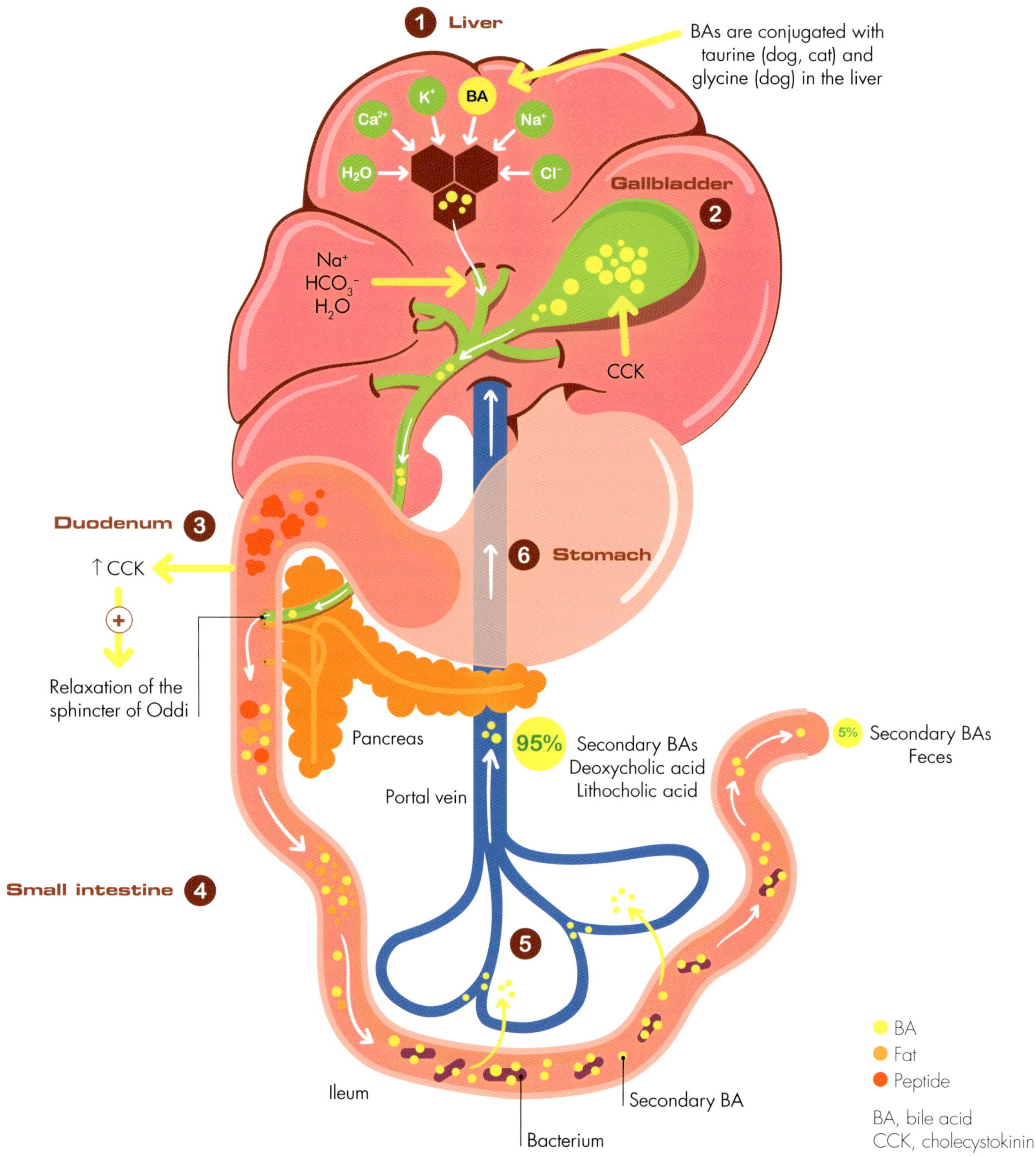

DISEASES OF THE GALLBLADDER AND BILE DUCTS

47 Cholecystitis

The term cholecystitis encompasses various inflammatory conditions of the gallbladder, but it is most often used to describe bacterial infections of the gallbladder (i.e., bacterial cholecystitis). Cholecystitis can also result from parasitic disease, biliary cancer, gallbladder mucoceles, cholelithiasis, and other poorly defined mechanisms (e.g., bile stasis). Although choleliths are identified in some patients, there is no evidence of a causal relationship. Cholecystitis may be either acute or chronic in nature, resulting in a wide range of clinical signs.

Clinical signs

- Mild cases are often asymptomatic.
- Anorexia.
- Vomiting.
- Abdominal pain.
- Chronic cases may have intermittent nonspecific clinical signs.

Diagnosis

- Clinical signs in conjunction with abdominal ultrasound findings:
  - Thickened gallbladder wall.
  - Pericholecystic steatitis.
- Cholecystocentesis to document bacteria in bacterial cholecystitis:
  - Cytology and culture.

62% of patients with cholecystitis have positive bacterial cultures. The most common isolates are *Escherichia coli*, *Enterococcus* spp., *Bacteroides* spp., *Streptococcus* spp., and *Clostridium* spp.

Anaphylaxis, pericardial effusion, and right-sided heart failure can result in gallbladder wall edema. However, these cases typically present with acute collapse or weakness.

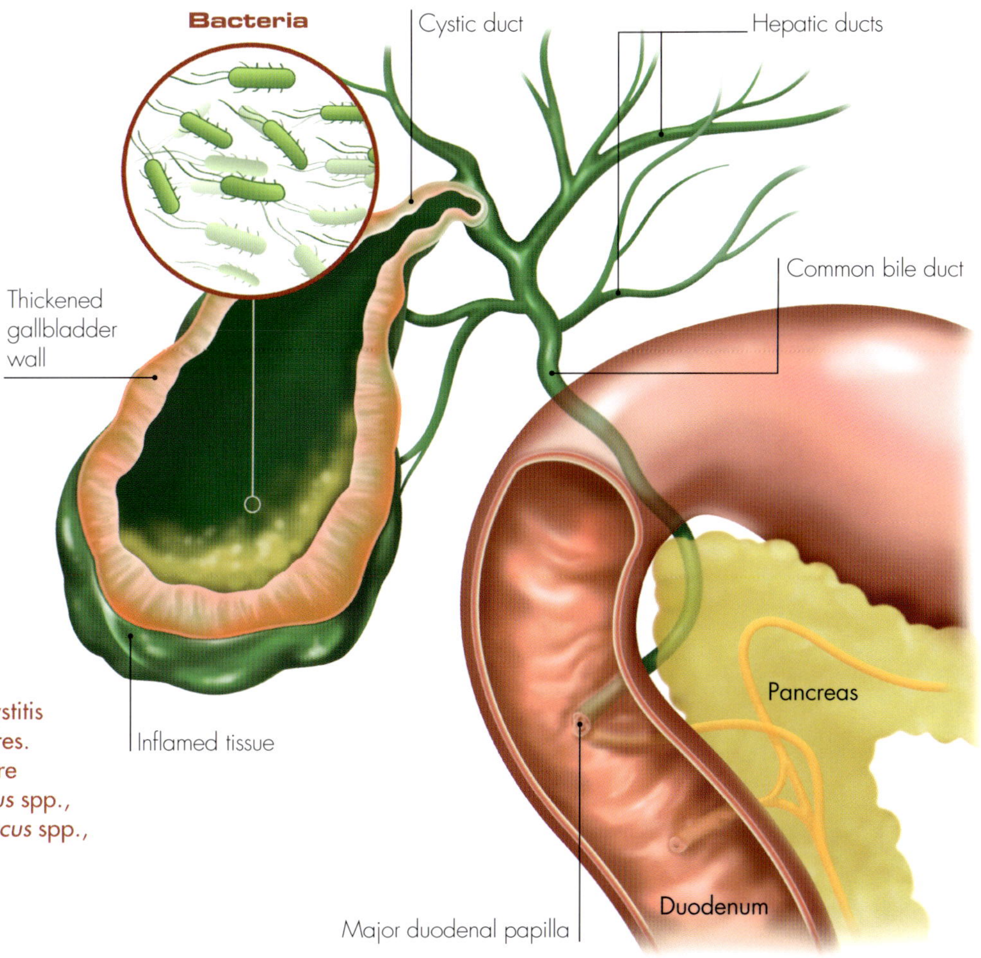

Treatment

- Medical management with intravenous fluids, analgesics, ursodeoxycholic acid, and antimicrobials. Antibiotics should be based on culture and sensitivity.
- Surgery is indicated when medical management fails or there is evidence of bile peritonitis.

Prognosis

- Generally good.
- Perioperative mortality rate: 20%–40%. The prognosis is excellent for patients that survive the postoperative period.

DISEASES OF THE GALLBLADDER AND BILE DUCTS

48 Gallbladder mucocele

A gallbladder mucocele occurs when the gallbladder distends abnormally from excessive accumulation of immobile semisolid mucoid material. This can lead to many complications, such as extrahepatic bile duct obstruction, cholecystitis, bile peritonitis, and pancreatitis. Shetland Sheepdogs, Cocker Spaniels, and Miniature Schnauzers are overrepresented. Although the exact mechanism by which gallbladder mucoceles form remains unknown, predisposing factors include dyslipidemia, dysmotility of the gallbladder, endocrine disease, and exogenous administration of corticosteroids.

Clinical signs

- Vomiting.
- Anorexia.
- Lethargy.
- Abdominal pain.
- Jaundice.
- Fever.

Dogs with gallbladder mucoceles can be asymptomatic to critically ill and in need of emergency surgery.

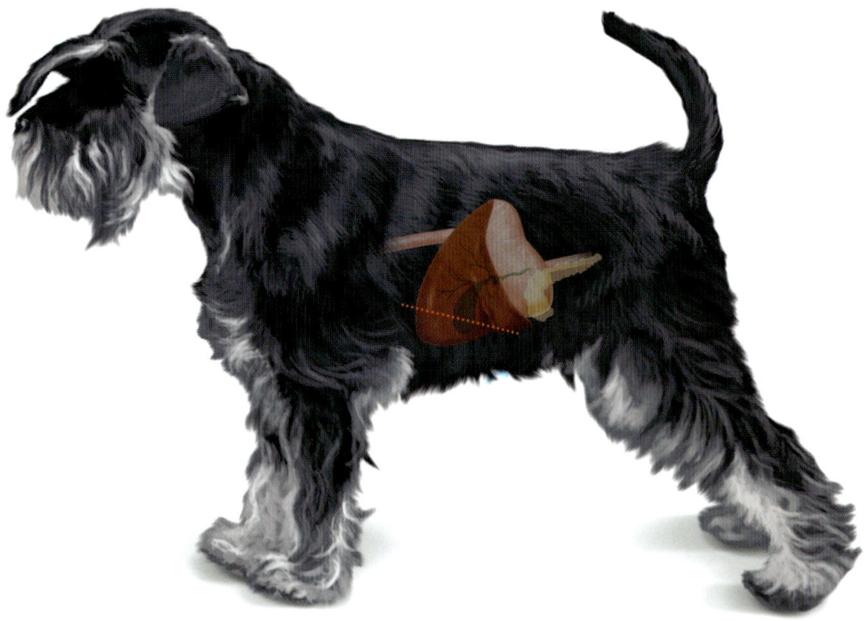

Diagnosis

- Abdominal ultrasound: distended gallbladder with immobile biliary sludge forming a stellate appearance (kiwifruit pattern).
- Biochemical changes may or may not be present and are indistinguishable from those of other hepatobiliary diseases.

Gallbladder mucocele progression

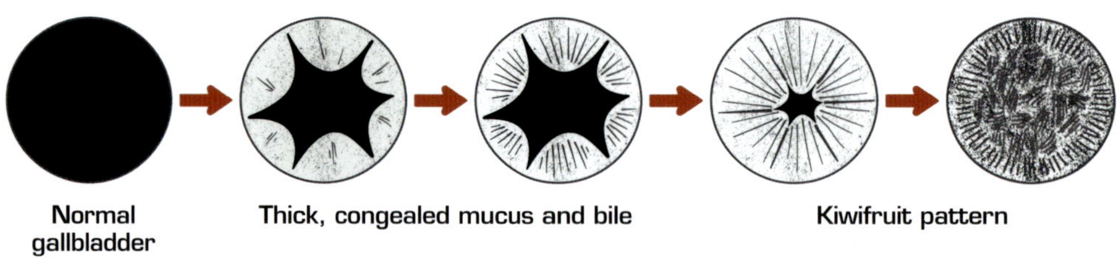

Treatment

- Surgery is indicated when there is concern of imminent rupture, obstruction, or bile peritonitis.
- In cases without rupture or obstruction, treatment with ursodeoxycholic acid, analgesia, and a low-fat diet may successfully resolve the clinical signs. Empirical antibiotics may also be indicated in patients with cranial abdominal pain or progressive increase in liver enzymes.
- Treatment of concurrent endocrine diseases (e.g., hypothyroidism, hyperadrenocorticism).

Prognosis

- Highly variable.
- Perioperative mortality rate: 20%–40%. The prognosis is excellent for patients that survive the perioperative period.
- Patients with septic and bile peritonitis carry the highest mortality rate.

DISEASES OF THE GALLBLADDER AND BILE DUCTS

49 Cholelithiasis and choledocholithiasis

Stones within the gallbladder are termed choleliths, while stones in the biliary ducts are termed choledocholiths. Cholesterol, bilirubin, and mixed choleliths have been reported in dogs and cats. Many patients are asymptomatic; however, in some cases, the gallbladder or bile duct may become obstructed or rupture. Older female dogs are predisposed, particularly those of the Miniature Schnauzer and Miniature Poodle breeds.

Clinical signs

- Patients may be asymptomatic to severely ill with signs of biliary obstruction or bile peritonitis.
- Abdominal pain.
- Vomiting.
- Anorexia.
- Jaundice.

Diagnosis

- Many stones are too small and are not mineralized enough to be seen on radiographs (14%–50% of choleliths can be seen).
- Abdominal ultrasound to visualize stones and evaluate the gallbladder and biliary tree.

Choleliths and choledocholiths are often found incidentally. Pancreatitis, gastroenteritis, and gastrointestinal foreign bodies may present with similar clinical signs and should be considered before attributing the signs to a gallstone.

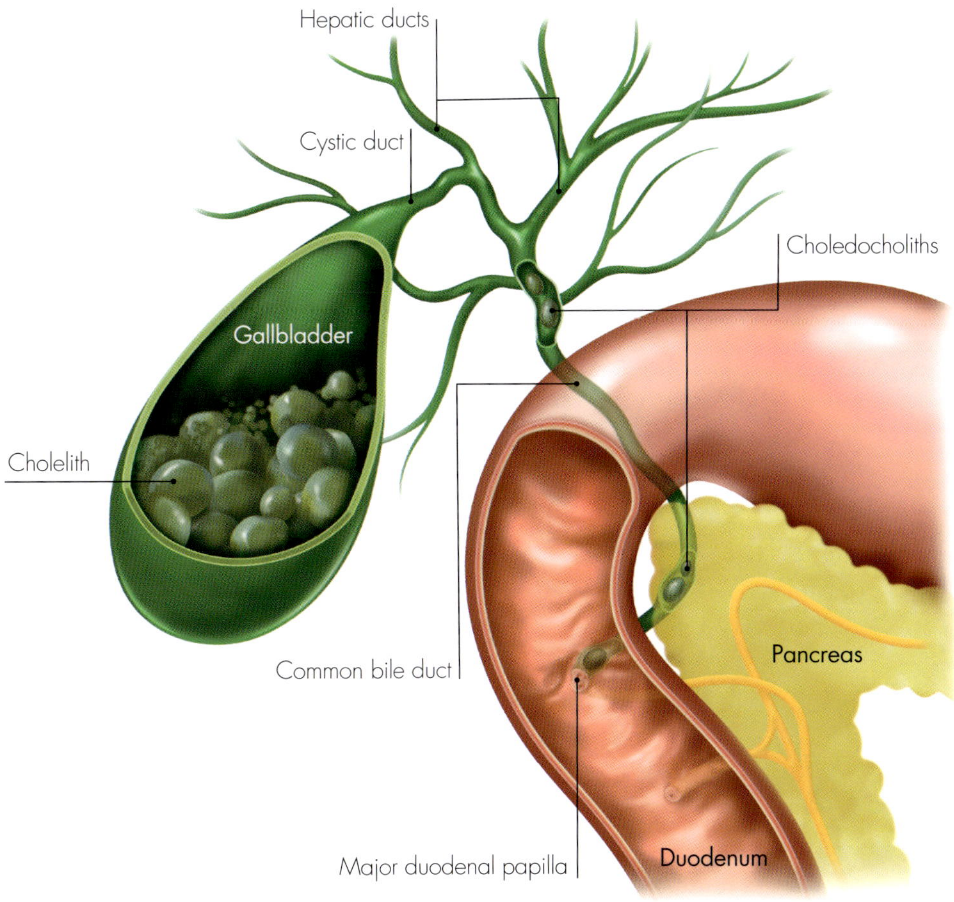

Treatment

- Most (53%–87%) stones are incidental findings and do not require intervention.
- Supportive care with intravenous fluids, ursodeoxycholic acid, analgesics, and antimicrobials may be considered in clinical patients with partial biliary obstruction.
- Surgery is indicated in cases with cholecystitis or biliary obstruction. Medical dissolution of stones in patients with severe acute obstruction is rarely successful.
- Treatment of concurrent endocrine diseases.

Prognosis

- Survival depends on the number and location of stones and the surgical procedure required.

DISEASES OF THE GALLBLADDER AND BILE DUCTS

50 Extrahepatic bile duct obstruction (EHBDO)

Blockage of normal bile flow to the gastrointestinal tract can be caused by many diseases, including cholelithiasis/choledocholithiasis, gallbladder mucoceles, cancer (e.g., biliary, hepatic, pancreatic), bile duct malformations, parasitic infection, extrinsic compression (e.g., enlarged lymph nodes, pancreatitis, pancreatic abscesses), duodenal foreign bodies, fibrosis (scar tissue formation secondary to peritonitis, trauma, pancreatitis, etc.), and bile duct strictures.

Clinical signs

- Anorexia.
- Vomiting.
- Abdominal pain.
- Fever.
- Jaundice.
- Complete obstruction may result in acholic (white) stools.

Diagnosis

- Serum biochemistry profile: elevated bilirubin, cholesterol, ALP, and/or GGT.
- Abdominal ultrasound.
- Exploratory laparotomy.

! Complete obstruction of the biliary system is a medical and surgical emergency.

! 20% of animals with EHBDO have cancer of the pancreas or bile duct.

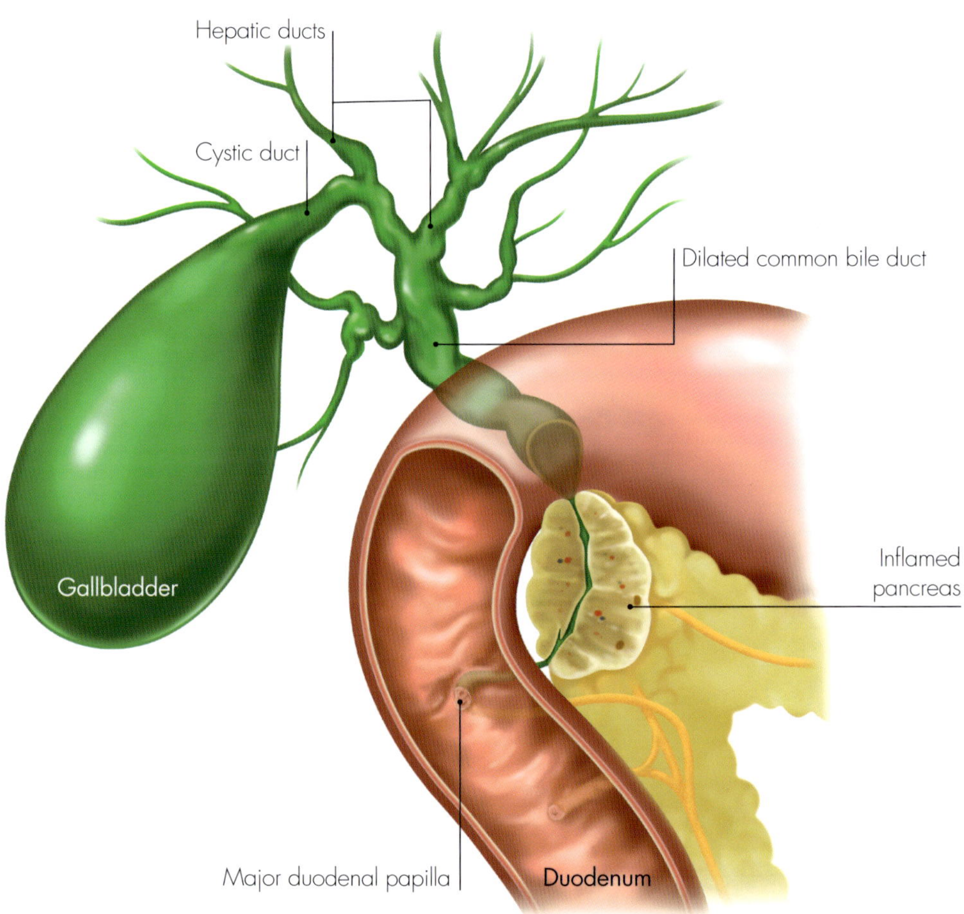

Treatment

- Dependent on the underlying cause. Pancreatitis-associated obstruction typically resolves as the acute pancreatitis subsides, whereas obstruction caused by cholelithiasis or cancer may require surgical intervention.
- Surgery may involve any combination of removal of masses, removal of portions of the pancreas or liver, placement of biliary stents, removal of the gallbladder, and diversion of the biliary system.

Prognosis

- When the underlying condition cannot be resolved, the prognosis is guarded to poor.
- Mortality rate in dogs: 28%–64%.
- Mortality rate in cats: 40% for noncancerous causes, 100% for cats with underlying cancer.

DISEASES OF THE GALLBLADDER AND BILE DUCTS

51 Biliary cancer

Primary cancer of the gallbladder or common bile duct is rare. Biliary cystadenomas, named for their cystic appearance, are benign tumors that account for more than 50% of feline hepatobiliary tumors. Biliary carcinomas are the most common malignant hepatobiliary tumor in cats and the second most common in dogs. They can be intrahepatic, extrahepatic, or within the gallbladder. Both solid and cystic carcinomas may occur.

Clinical signs

- Nonspecific signs (e.g., anorexia, vomiting).
- Jaundice.
- Signs of biliary duct obstruction may be present (see Sheet 50).

Diagnosis

- Serum biochemistry profile may reveal elevated bilirubin, cholesterol, ALP, and/or GGT.
- Abdominal ultrasound or CT scan.

Biliary carcinomas are more common in female dogs and dogs that are 10 years of age or older. Biliary cystadenomas are more common in male cats.

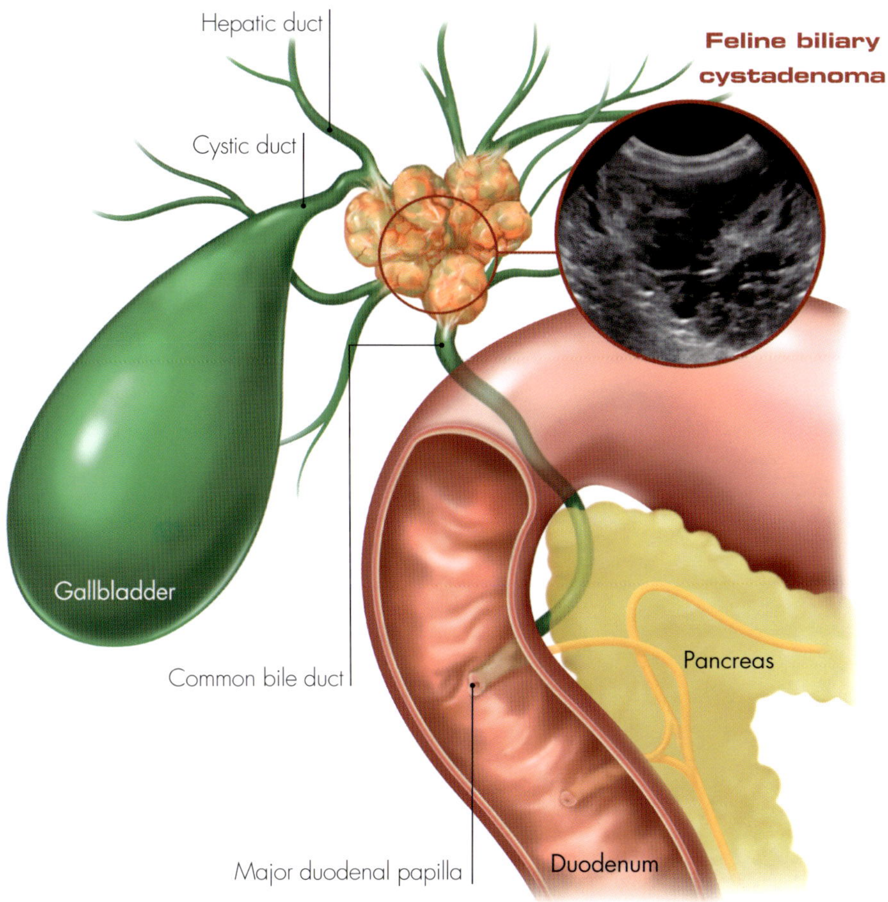

Treatment

- Surgical excision when possible. Liver lobectomy is recommended for patients with single biliary masses or multifocal lesions confined to one or two lobes.

Prognosis

- Biliary cystadenomas typically do not cause clinical signs until they are large enough to compress nearby organs. The prognosis is very good following surgical resection.
- Biliary carcinomas have an aggressive behavior. Metastasis occurs in 88% of dogs (lymph nodes, lungs) and 67%–90% of cats (diffuse metastasis within the abdomen, i.e., carcinomatosis). Most patients die within 6 months of liver lobectomy due to local recurrence and metastatic disease.

DISEASES OF THE LIVER

52 Congenital portosystemic shunt (cPSS)

A cPSS is a birth defect characterized by an anomalous vessel that bypasses blood delivery to the liver. It can course through the liver (intrahepatic) or outside the liver (extrahepatic).

Normal

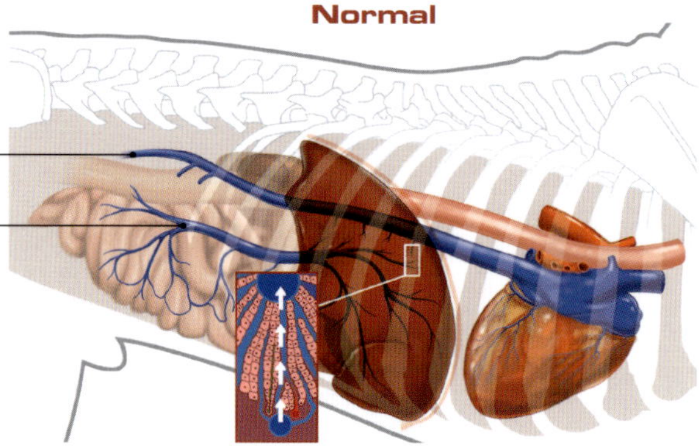

Most dogs and cats with cPSS have clinical signs before 1–2 years of age.

Clinical signs

- Failure to thrive.
- Finicky appetite, intermittent vomiting/diarrhea.
- Increased thirst or urination or signs of urinary disease from bladder stones.
- Behavior changes.

Diagnosis

- Complete blood count may reveal a mild to moderate microcytic, normochromic anemia.
- Serum biochemistry profile often reveals decreased liver function.
- Elevated bile acids.
- Imaging to confirm the presence and type of cPSS:
  - Abdominal ultrasound or CT scan.
  - Portovenography.
  - Scintigraphy (gold standard).

Extrahepatic cPSS

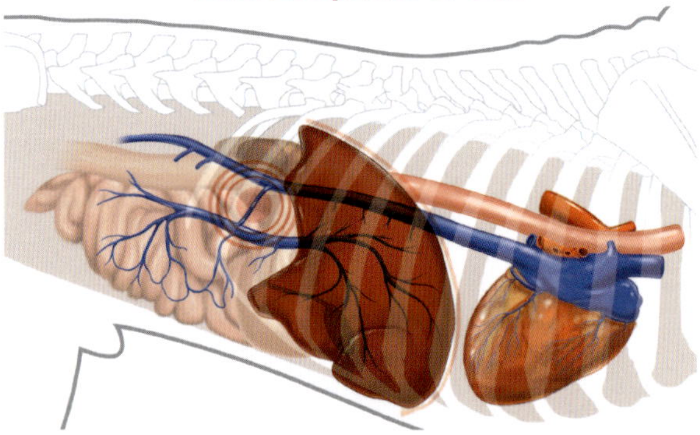

Intrahepatic cPSS

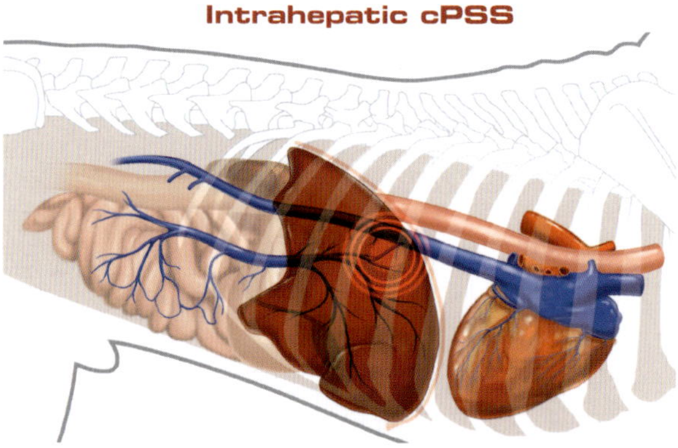

Treatment

- Medical management:
  - Hepatic encephalopathy: moderately protein-restricted diet and oral lactulose ± antibiotics (metronidazole, neomycin).
  - Nonbenzodiazepine anti-seizure drugs (e.g., levetiracetam) if seizures.
- Surgery, after medical stabilization, is the treatment of choice:
  - Extrahepatic cPSS: gradual occlusion devices (e.g., ameroid constrictors, cellophane bands).
  - Intrahepatic cPSS: percutaneous transvenous coil embolization.

Prognosis

- Medical management alone can be successful in extrahepatic cPSS patients with mild to moderate clinical signs. It is not recommended for intrahepatic cPSS.
- Surgery:
  - Extrahepatic cPSS: 90%–95% survival rate. Good prognosis.
  - Intrahepatic cPSS: 23%–64% mortality rate. Fair prognosis.

DISEASES OF THE LIVER

53 Hepatic arteriovenous malformation (HAVM)

HAVM is a rare condition whereby numerous small communications occur between high-pressure arteries and low-pressure veins. Most often, a branch of the hepatic artery communicates directly with the portal vein via dozens to hundreds of aberrant shunting vessels. Blood, moving from high to low pressure, dumps into the portal vein, overwhelming it. Portal hypertension (increased pressure in the vein that carries blood from the abdominal organs to the liver) leads to the formation of multiple extrahepatic shunts to decompress the system. HAVMs are most often diagnosed in young dogs, and less commonly in cats.

Clinical signs

- Ascites is very common (75%).
- Signs of hepatic encephalopathy (changes in behavior, staring into space, circling, seizures).
- Vomiting, diarrhea.
- Stunted growth, lethargy.
- Heart murmurs (20%).

Diagnosis

- CT angiography.

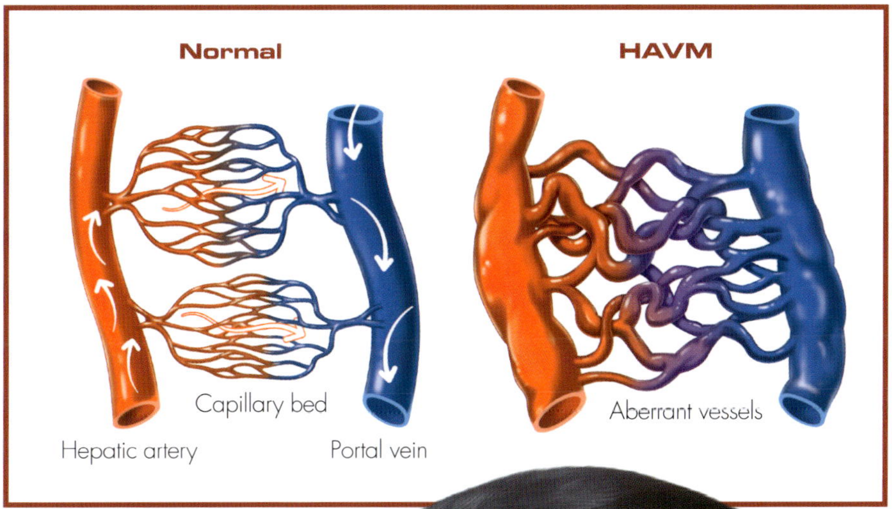

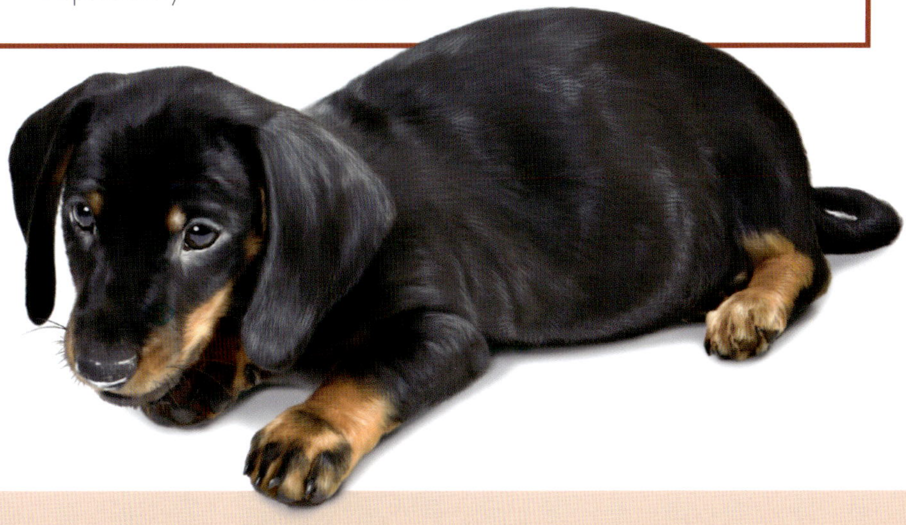

Most affected animals are diagnosed within the first year of life, and clinical signs are associated with multiple acquired extrahepatic portosystemic shunts or ascites.

Treatment

- Glue embolization under fluoroscopic guidance.
- Liver lobectomy if the changes are confined to one or two lobes.
- Proton pump inhibitors (omeprazole) in case of gastrointestinal ulceration secondary to portal hypertension.
- Medical management of congenital portosystemic shunts (see Sheet 52).

Prognosis

- Generally good in dogs undergoing glue embolization with or without liver lobectomy.
- Fair to good long-term outcome in dogs treated with surgery alone (38%–57% survival).

75% of dogs require lifelong dietary and medical management of clinical signs due to acquired extrahepatic portosystemic shunts.

DISEASES OF THE LIVER

54 Canine acute hepatitis

Acute hepatitis in dogs can be caused by toxins, chemicals, medications, infections, and ischemia.

Clinical signs

- Acute onset.
- Anorexia, vomiting, diarrhea.
- Fever.
- Abdominal pain.
- Increased thirst and urination.
- Jaundice.

Diagnosis

- Based on complete blood count, chemistry profile, clinical findings, and history.
- Marked elevation in serum liver enzymes (ALT often greater than ALP).
- Evidence of liver dysfunction (e.g., hypoalbuminemia, hypocholesterolemia, hypoglycemia, low BUN, prolonged clotting times) may or may not be present.
- Testing for leptospirosis and other regionally relevant infectious diseases.
- Abdominal ultrasound.
- Cholecystocentesis for bile cytology and culture.
- Liver biopsy may be necessary.

Acute hepatitis can be rapidly fatal, completely reversible, or progress to chronic hepatitis. Early recognition and intervention are key to a successful outcome.

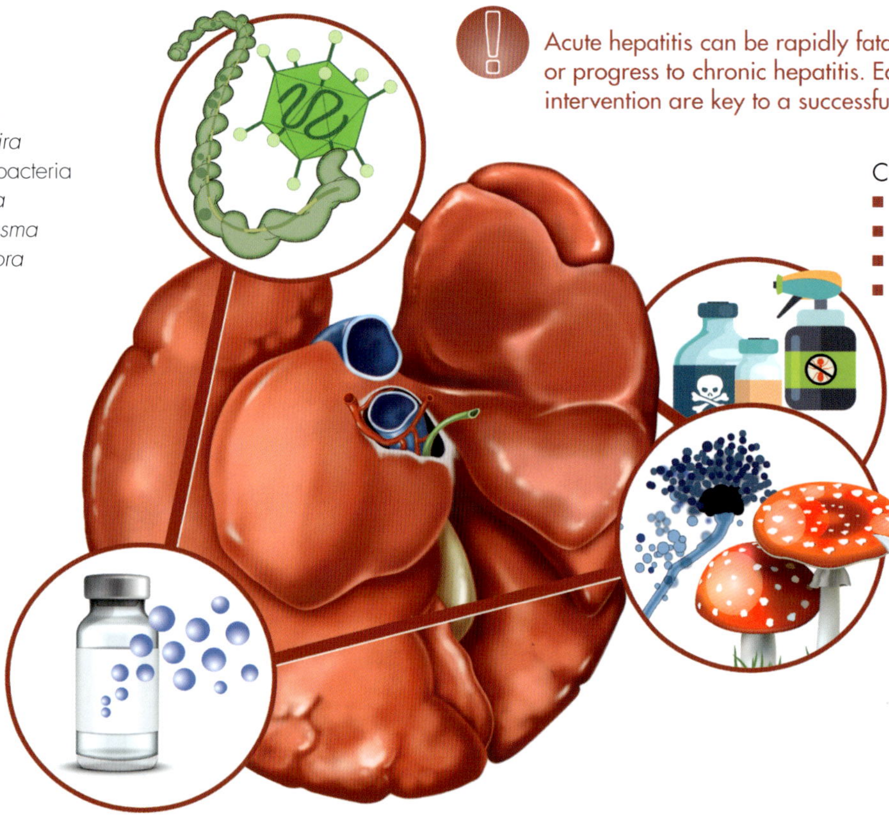

Infections
- CAdV-1
- *Leptospira*
- Enteric bacteria
- *Ehrlichia*
- *Toxoplasma*
- *Neospora*
- Sepsis

Chemicals
- Heavy metals
- Carbon tetrachloride
- Pine oil
- Chlorinated hydrocarbons

Medications
- Phenobarbital
- NSAIDs
- Acetaminophen
- Azathioprine
- Azoles
- Tetracyclines
- Chemotherapeutics (e.g., lomustine)

Toxins
- *Amanita* mushrooms
- Mycotoxins (e.g., aflatoxins)
- Blue-green algae
- Sago palms
- Xylitol (artificial sweetener)

Treatment

- Activated charcoal if recent exposure to a known hepatotoxin that undergoes enterohepatic recirculation.
- Hospitalization, intravenous fluids, nutritional support, and close monitoring.
- Antioxidants: N-acetylcysteine or S-adenosylmethionine.
- Antibiotics based on suspected infectious cause.
- Treatment of hepatic encephalopathy if present (see Sheet 52).
- Dextrose supplementation in case of hypoglycemia.
- Subcutaneous or oral vitamin K_1 if prolonged clotting times.

Prognosis

- Highly variable depending on the underlying cause and how quickly appropriate therapy is instituted.
- 30% of cases progress to chronic hepatitis.

Vaccination against leptospirosis should be considered for dogs in high-risk areas.

DISEASES OF THE LIVER

55 Vacuolar hepatopathy

Vacuolar hepatopathy is characterized by the accumulation of fat or glycogen in vacuoles (small fluid-filled cavities) within hepatocytes. As a result, liver cells swell and the liver enlarges (hepatomegaly).

Vacuolar hepatopathy is common in dogs. Because it can be difficult to determine the underlying cause, much of the diagnosis involves evaluating for and ruling out potential causes.

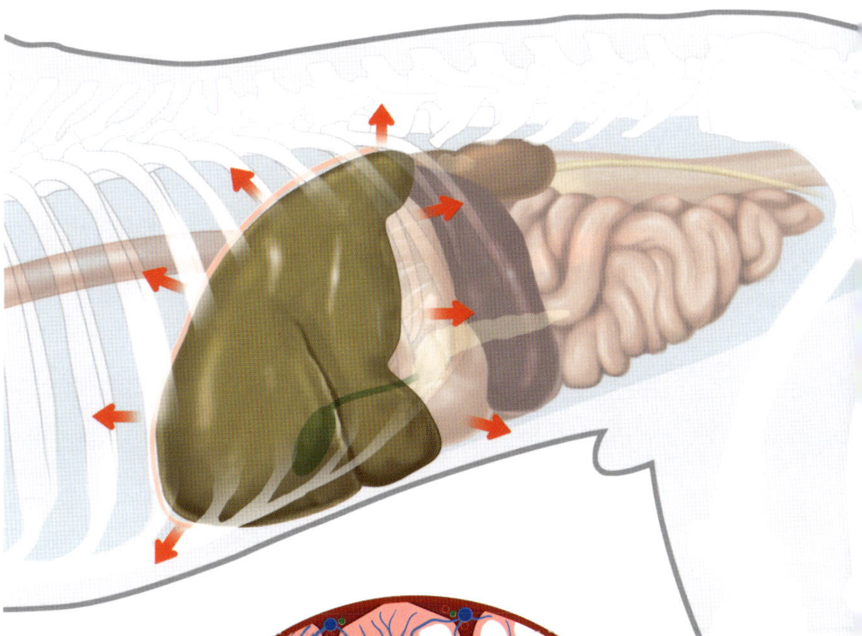

Causes

- Exogenous corticosteroids (dogs).
- Endocrine diseases (e.g., hyperadrenocorticism, hypothyroidism, diabetes mellitus).
- Hyperlipidemia.
- Toxicoses (e.g., aflatoxin in dogs, vitamin A in cats).
- Vacuolar hepatopathy of Scottish Terriers.
- Hepatocutaneous syndrome (see Sheet 59).
- Feline hepatic lipidosis (see Sheet 63).
- Secondary to another disease (e.g., heart disease, cancer, gastrointestinal disease, kidney disease, infections, other hepatobiliary diseases).

Clinical signs

- Hepatomegaly; often hyperechoic liver on ultrasound.
- ALP often greater than ALT.
- Clinical signs related to the underlying cause.

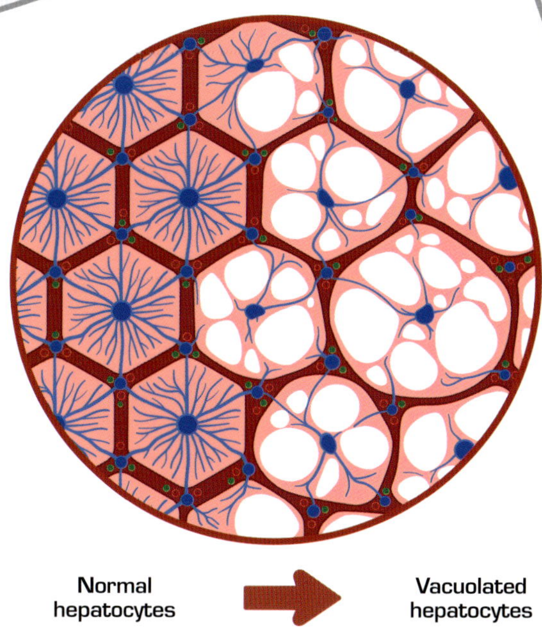

Diagnosis

- Discontinuation of medications and herbal supplements.
- Thyroid and hyperadrenocorticism testing.
- Fasting triglycerides.
- Screen for other underlying diseases (e.g., imaging).
- Liver biopsy.

Treatment

- Treatment of underlying causes.

Prognosis

- Often benign and reversible, but some causes may be progressive.
- Scottish Terriers get a unique and progressive form of vacuolar hepatopathy that increases the risk of hepatocellular carcinoma.

DISEASES OF THE LIVER

56 Canine chronic hepatitis

The cause of canine chronic hepatitis is often unknown, but considerations include copper accumulation, medications (e.g., phenobarbital, NSAIDs), infectious diseases (e.g., leptospirosis, tick-borne diseases, mycobacterial, fungal, protozoal), breed-specific hepatopathies (e.g., Cocker Spaniels, Labradors), and progression of an episode of acute hepatitis.

Clinical signs

- Decreased appetite, weight loss.
- Lethargy.
- Vomiting, diarrhea.
- Excessive thirst and urination.
- Ascites.
- Jaundice.
- Signs of hepatic encephalopathy.

Diagnosis

- Serum biochemistry profile, coagulation times, bile acids, and fasting ammonia to evaluate liver function.
- Abdominal ultrasound.
- CT scan to evaluate for acquired portosystemic shunts.
- Liver biopsy for histology, culture, and copper quantification.

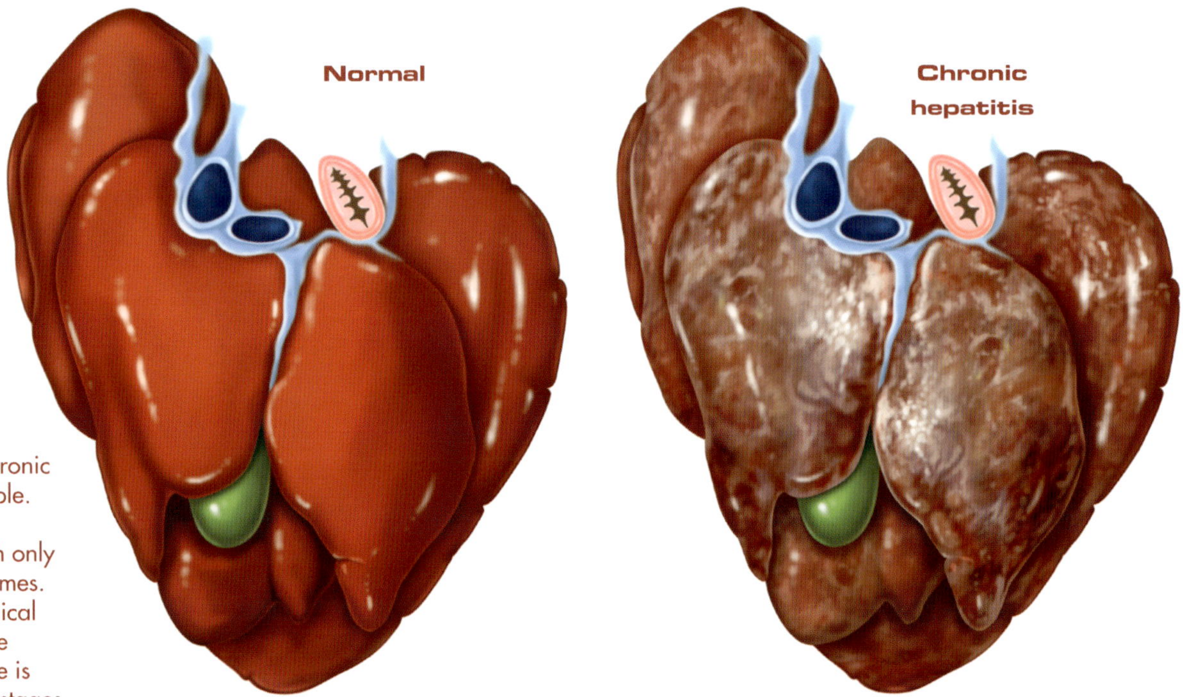

Clinical signs of chronic hepatitis are variable. Initially, dogs are asymptomatic, with only elevated liver enzymes. However, once clinical signs of liver failure appear, the disease is often in advanced stages.

Treatment

- Treatment of the underlying cause when possible.
- S-adenosylmethionine with or without silybin.
- Ursodeoxycholic acid.
- Antibiotics based on culture and sensitivity.
- Treatment of hepatic encephalopathy if present (see Sheet 52).
- Oral or subcutaneous vitamin K_1 if prolonged clotting times.
- After ruling out other causes, immunosuppressants (e.g., prednisone, cyclosporine) for idiopathic chronic hepatitis.

Prognosis

- Median survival: 18–36 months.
- Prognosis is poor (1–2 months) if cirrhosis or lobular dissecting hepatitis are diagnosed.
- Hyperbilirubinemia, prolonged clotting times, hypoalbuminemia, ascites, and the degree of fibrosis on biopsy are associated with a poor prognosis.

DISEASES OF THE LIVER

57 Copper-associated hepatopathy

Copper associated-hepatopathy may occur in any breed, but the Bedlington Terrier, Dalmatian, Labrador Retriever, Doberman Pinscher, and West Highland White Terrier are predisposed. Copper accumulation is thought to occur secondary to genetic mutations resulting in altered elimination of copper in the liver. Increased amount and bioavailability of copper in commercial dog foods may also be a contributing factor in at-risk breeds. Accumulation of copper within liver cells results in oxidative stress, cell death, and inflammation.

Clinical signs

- Decreased appetite, weight loss.
- Lethargy.
- Vomiting, diarrhea.
- Excessive thirst and urination.
- Ascites.
- Jaundice.
- Signs of hepatic encephalopathy.

Diagnosis

- Serum biochemistry profile, coagulation times, bile acids, and/or fasting ammonia to evaluate liver function.
- Abdominal ultrasound.
- CT scan to evaluate for acquired portosystemic shunts.
- Liver biopsy for histology, culture, and copper quantification:
  - Centrilobular copper accumulation.
  - Copper >1000 µg/g dry weight liver.

Clinical signs can vary from asymptomatic, with only elevated liver enzymes, to signs of liver failure.

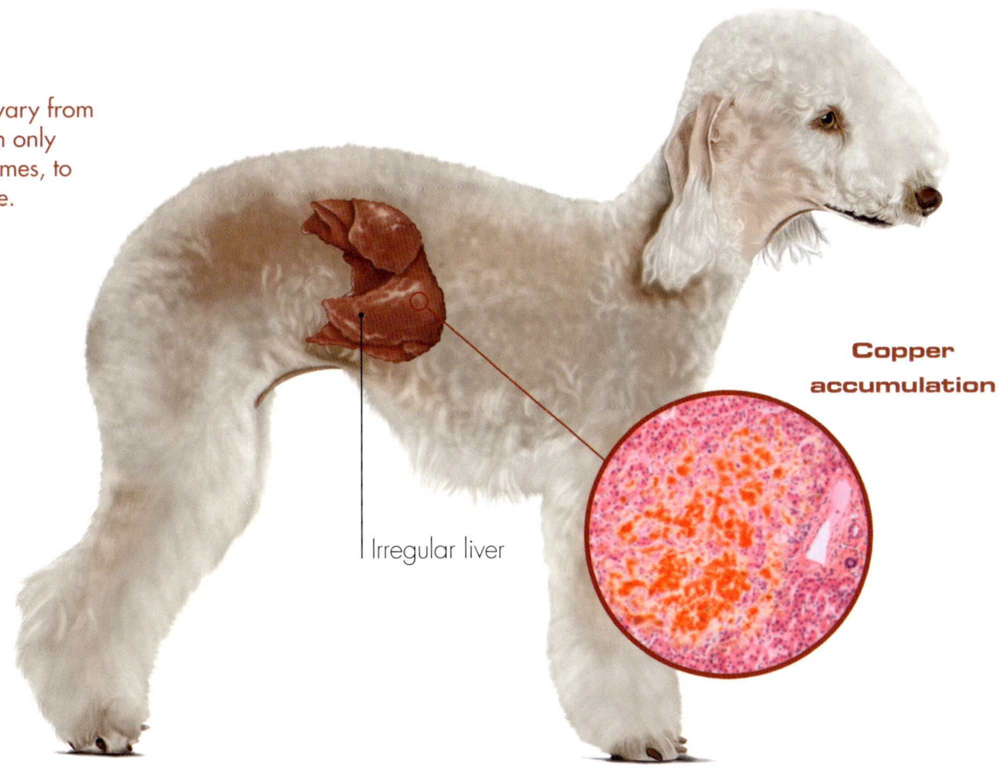

Treatment

- Treatment of chronic hepatitis (see Sheet 56).
- Low-copper diet.
- Administration of a copper chelator (e.g., pencillamine, trientine) for 3–6 months, ideally based on resolution of copper accumulation on liver biopsy.
- Esophageal feeding tubes help provide nutritional support and facilitate medication administration.

Prognosis

- Can be good with early diagnosis and intervention.
- Dogs with end-stage liver disease and signs of decompensated liver function have a poorer prognosis.

DISEASES OF THE LIVER

58 Cirrhosis

Cirrhosis is the end-stage consequence of liver inflammation secondary to chronic liver disease, drugs, or toxins. In cirrhosis, nonfunctional fibrous scar tissue replaces functional liver tissue, resulting in a small and irregular liver.

Clinical signs

- Jaundice.
- Ascites.
- Anorexia, vomiting, and/or diarrhea.
- Signs of hepatic encephalopathy.

Diagnosis

- Biochemical parameters show evidence of liver failure (low BUN, albumin, cholesterol, and glucose; elevated total bilirubin, bile acids, and ammonia).
- Small, nodular, irregular liver.
- Multiple acquired portosystemic shunts may be seen on ultrasound or CT scan.
- Although biopsy is necessary for a definitive diagnosis, the limitations of sampling error and poor prognosis result in diagnosis often being based on imaging and clinicopathologic parameters.

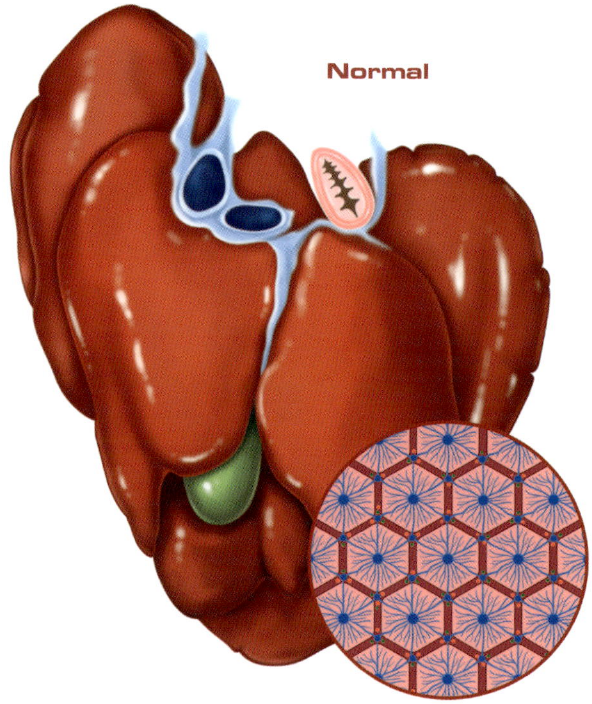

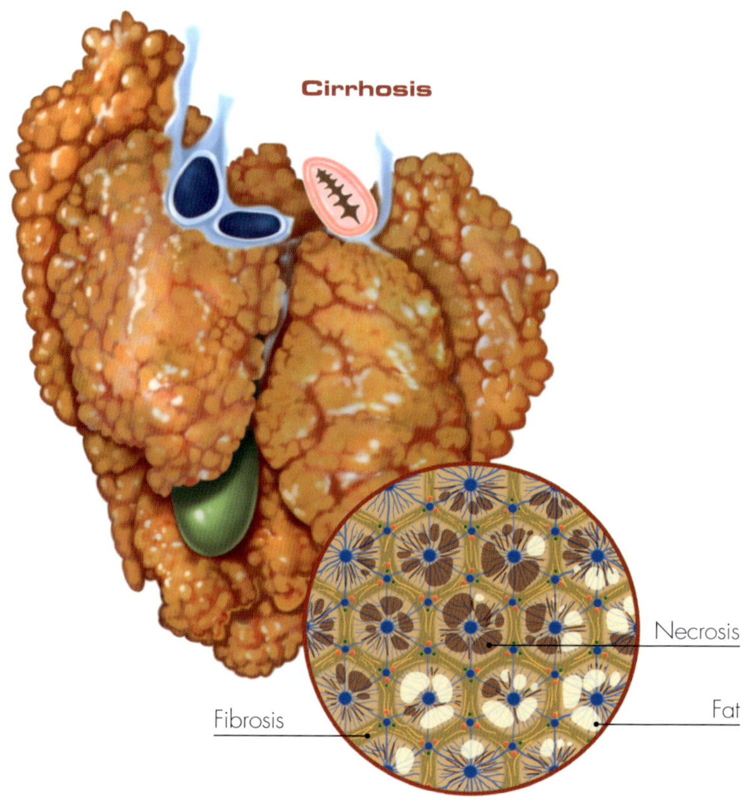

Treatment

- Treatment of the underlying chronic hepatopathy if possible.
- Management of hepatic encephalopathy (see Sheet 52).
- Management of ascites with diuretics (e.g., spironolactone).

Prognosis

- Poor.

By the time clinical signs of cirrhosis are detected, less than 20% of functional liver tissue remains. As a result, the prognosis is poor.

DISEASES OF THE LIVER

59 Hepatocutaneous syndrome

Hepatocutaneous syndrome is a rare, chronic, progressive liver disease in dogs characterized by hyperkeratotic, erythematous crusting lesions on the paw pads, nose, and periorbital and perianal regions.

Clinical signs

- Crusting and exudative lesions on the paw pads and periocular, perioral, and genital regions.
- Lameness and reluctance to walk due to paw pad lesions.
- Decreased appetite.
- Signs of diabetes mellitus may be present (excessive thirst and urination, weight loss).

Diagnosis

- Biochemistry panel: predominately cholestatic pattern (ALP greater than ALT).
- Liver ultrasound: unique "honeycomb" or "Swiss Cheese" pattern.
- Liver biopsy: vacuolar hepatopathy. It is not specific for a diagnosis.
- Skin biopsy for definitive diagnosis.

Concurrent diabetes mellitus occurs in 25%–40% of dogs with hepatocutaneous syndrome.

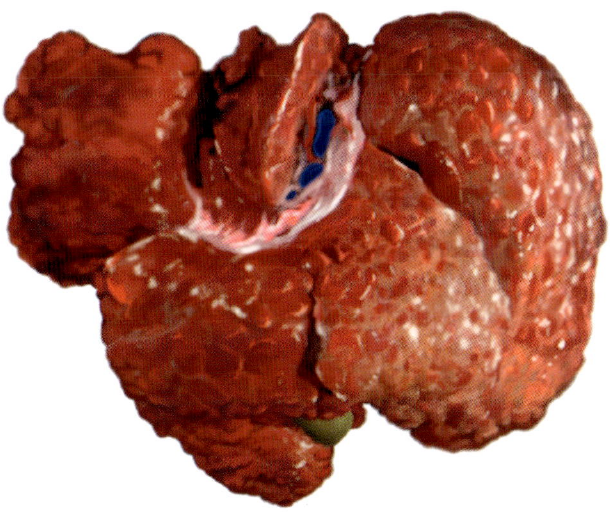

Hyperkeratotic paw pad

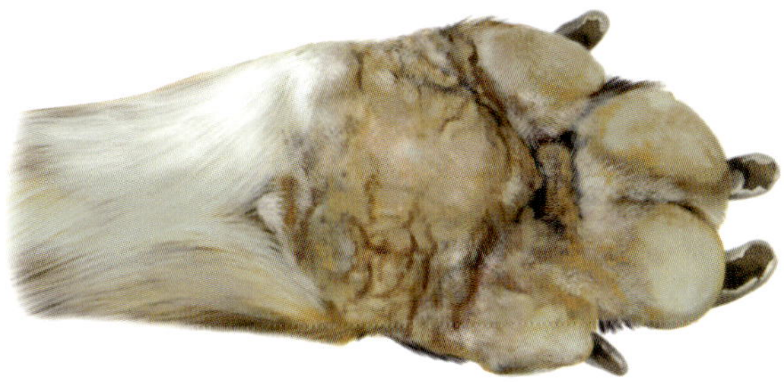

Hyperkeratotic nose

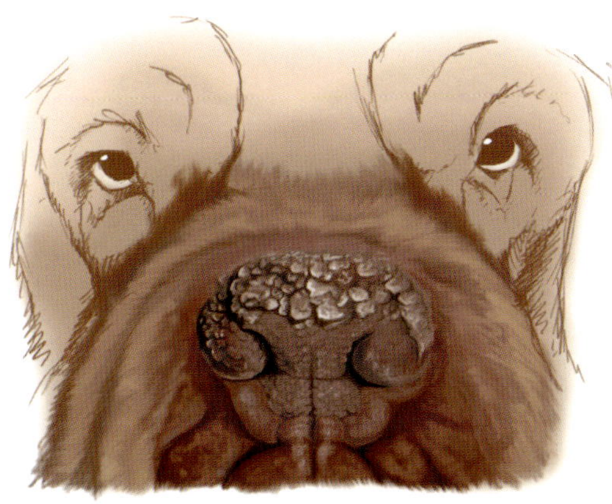

Treatment

- Intravenous amino acid infusions every 1–2 weeks and then as needed to control clinical signs.
- Targeted nutritional intervention including oral amino acid supplements and S-adenosylmethionine.
- Other considerations: zinc methionine, omega-3 fatty acids (DHA + EPA).
- Prompt treatment of secondary bacterial infections.

Prognosis

- Without aggressive intervention, most dogs survive less than 6 months.
- Long-term survival (>4.9 years) is possible with a combination of intravenous amino acid infusions and targeted nutritional intervention.

DISEASES OF THE LIVER

60 Feline neutrophilic cholangitis

Neutrophilic cholangitis is characterized by the presence of neutrophils within the lumen and/or epithelium of the bile ducts. It is suspected to be caused by ascending bacterial infections from the intestine.

Clinical signs

- Anorexia, weight loss.
- Vomiting.
- Abdominal pain.

Diagnosis

- Abdominal radiographic and ultrasonographic findings are nonspecific.
- Cholecystocentesis for bile cytology and culture.
- Liver biopsy: neutrophilic infiltrates.
- Culture and sensitivity of liver tissue to guide antibiotic decisions.

Cats with neutrophilic cholangitis are often anorexic and at risk of developing secondary hepatic lipidosis.

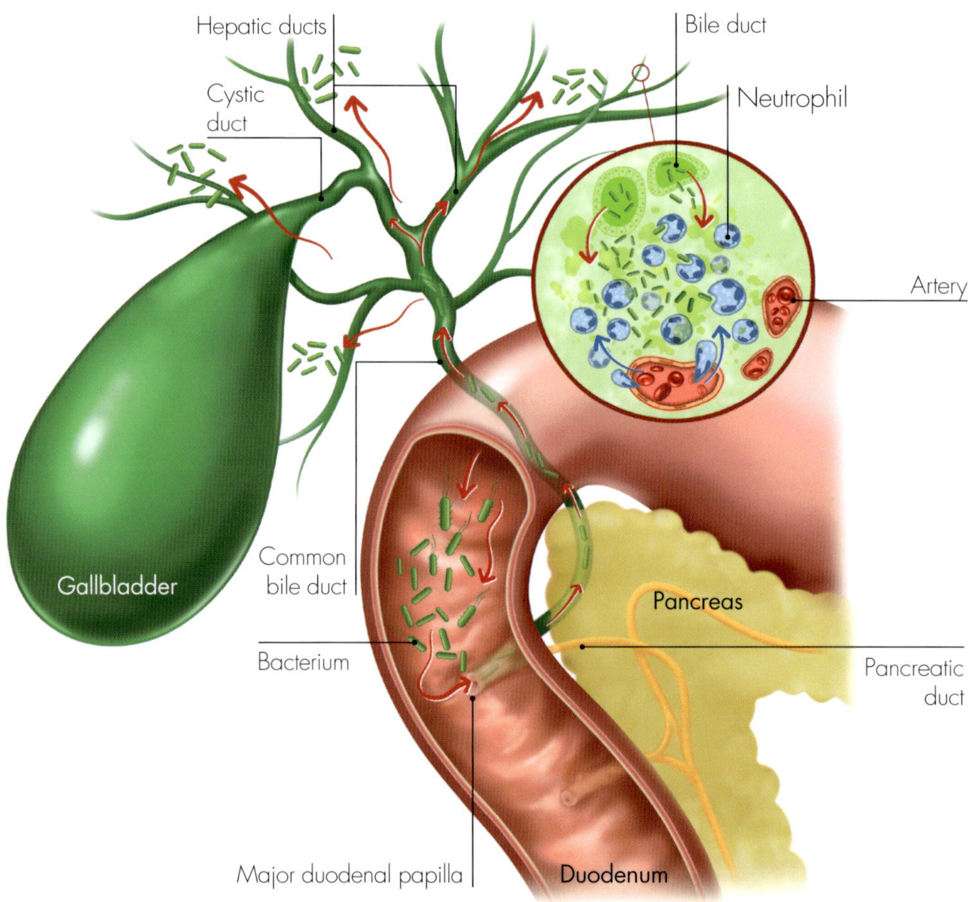

In cats, the common bile duct and pancreatic duct open into the duodenum through one opening, unlike in dogs, where they enter separately. Reflux of bacteria-rich duodenal juice into these ducts is thought to play a role in the development of neutrophilic cholangitis.

Treatment

- Medical management with intravenous fluids, analgesics, ursodeoxycholic acid, and antibiotics (4–8 weeks) based on culture and sensitivity results when possible.
- Esophageal feeding tubes help provide nutritional support and facilitate medication administration.
- Surgical intervention may be required for cats that develop extrahepatic bile duct obstruction secondary to neutrophilic inflammation.

Prognosis

- Generally good.
- Cats with secondary extrahepatic bile duct obstruction have a poorer prognosis.

Antibiotics are the primary therapy for neutrophilic cholangitis

DISEASES OF THE LIVER

61 Feline lymphocytic cholangitis

Lymphocytic cholangitis is characterized by the infiltration of lymphocytes within the portal areas of the hepatic lobules, which may be associated with fibrosis and bile duct hyperplasia. The cause remains unknown, but this disease is thought to result from an immune-mediated or infectious phenomenon. Similar to neutrophilic cholangitis, concurrent inflammatory bowel disease and pancreatitis are common in cats with lymphocytic cholangitis.

Clinical signs

- Clinical signs may be chronic and intermittent.
- Dysorexia (abnormal appetite or change in food-seeking behavior).
- Weight loss.
- Vomiting.
- Jaundice.

Diagnosis

- Abdominal radiographic and ultrasonographic findings are nonspecific.
- Cholecystocentesis for bile cytology and culture.
- Liver biopsy for culture and histopathology: lymphocytic infiltrates near the portal areas.

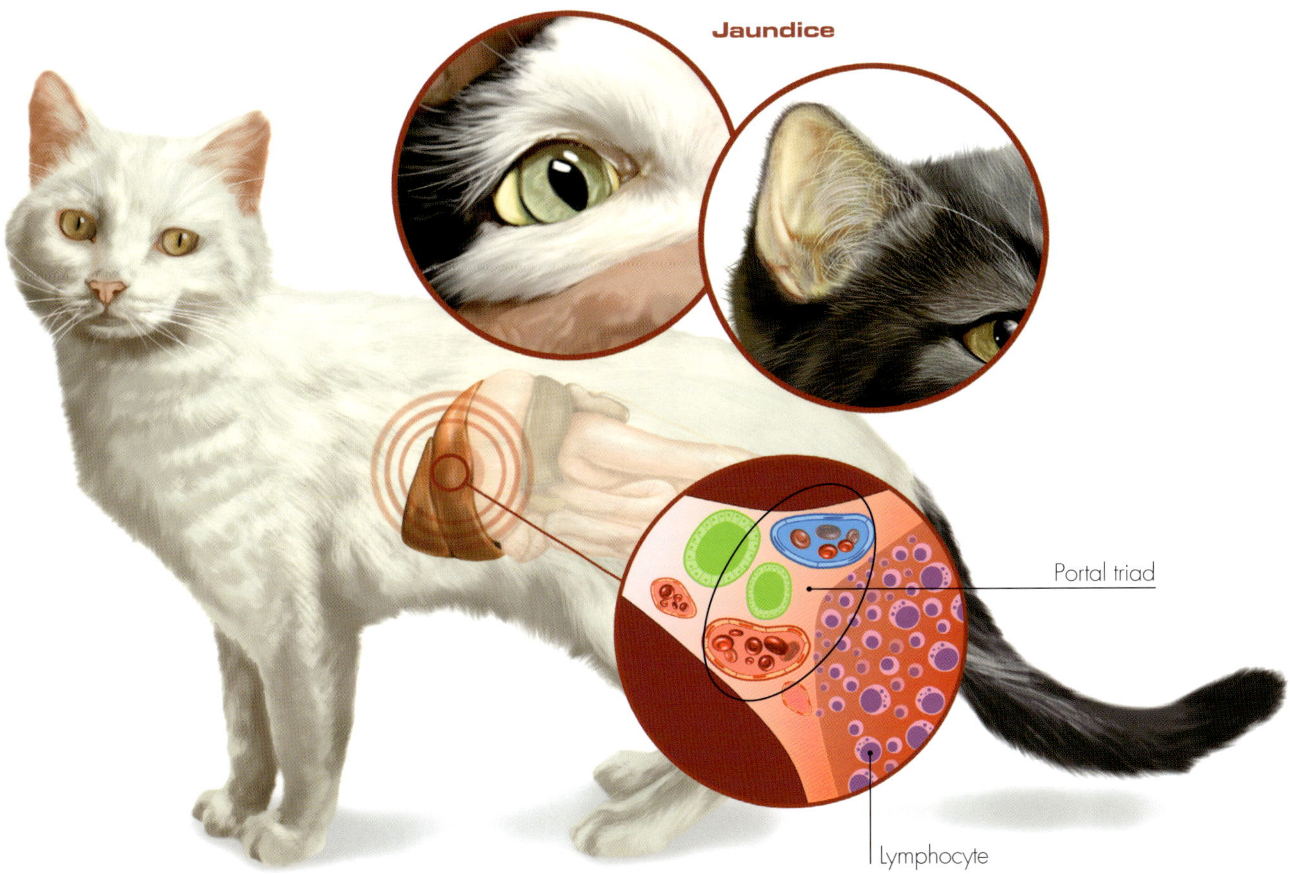

Treatment

- Medical management with intravenous fluids, analgesics, and hepatoprotectants (e.g., S-adenosylmethionine).
- Broad-spectrum antibiotics while awaiting results of bacterial cultures. They may be discontinued if cultures are negative.
- Immunosuppression with prednisolone.

Prognosis

- Generally good. Some cats may not respond to treatment.
- Lifelong management and monitoring are required.

Immunosuppression with prednisolone is the mainstay of treatment for lymphocytic cholangitis.

DISEASES OF THE LIVER

62 Feline triaditis

Triaditis is characterized by inflammation of the intestines (inflammatory bowel disease), pancreas (pancreatitis), and bile ducts (cholangitis). The cholangitis seen in triaditis may be lymphocytic or neutrophilic, such that both infectious and immune-mediated causes can play a role.

Clinical signs

- Clinical signs may be chronic and intermittent.
- Dysorexia, weight loss.
- Vomiting, diarrhea.
- Jaundice.

Diagnosis

- Abdominal ultrasound may reveal pancreatitis, intestinal wall thickening, loss of intestinal layering, and enlargement of abdominal lymph nodes.
- Cholecystocentesis for bile cytology and culture.
- Serum cobalamin, folate, fPLI, and TLI.
- Biopsy of the liver, gastrointestinal tract, and pancreas for definitive diagnosis.

In cats, the common bile duct and pancreatic duct open into the duodenum through one opening, unlike in dogs, where they enter separately. Reflux of bacteria-rich duodenum juice into these ducts is thought to result in feline triaditis.

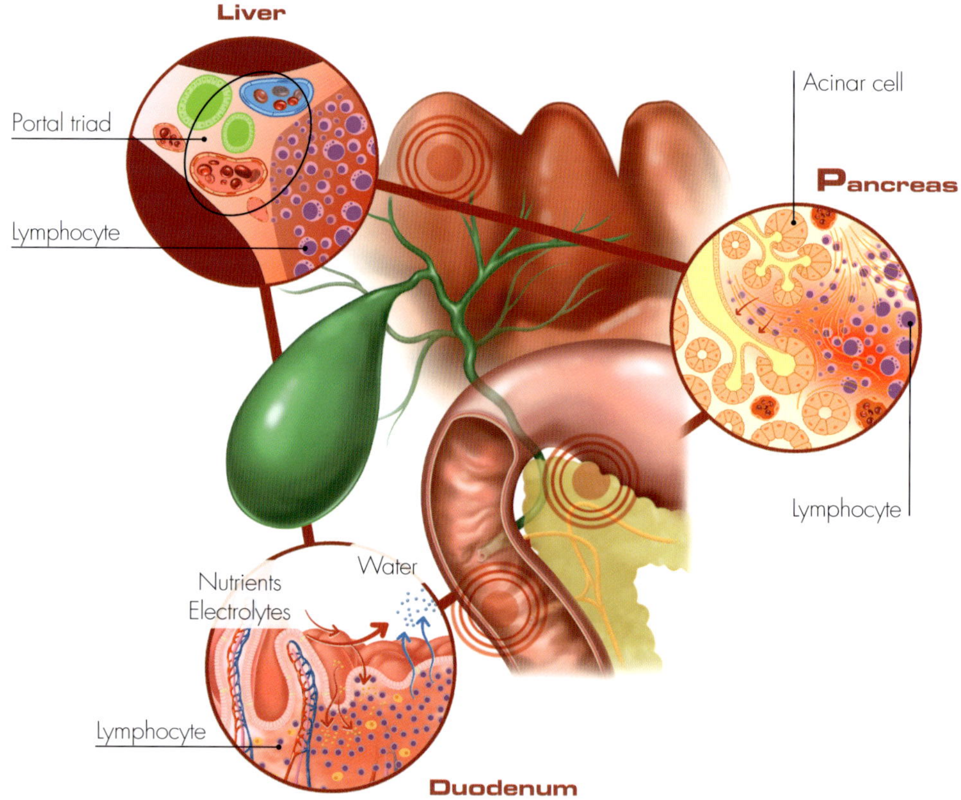

Most cats with triaditis have a normal liver on ultrasound.

Treatment

- Diet trial (hydrolyzed or novel protein).
- Supportive care with antinausea, appetite-stimulating, and pain medications. Esophageal feeding tubes provide consistent nutrition and help with medication administration.
- Hepatoprotectants (e.g., S-adenosylmethionine, ursodeoxycholic acid).
- Antibiotics based on culture and sensitivity.
- Cobalamin supplementation.
- Immunosuppression with prednisolone if there is no response to dietary trial and antibiotics.

Prognosis

- Good in most cats with mild disease.
- Cats with systemic complications (low blood pressure, hepatic encephalopathy, coagulopathy) may have a poor prognosis and warrant aggressive therapy.
- Low serum albumin and glucose are associated with a poorer prognosis.

DISEASES OF THE LIVER

63 Feline hepatic lipidosis

Hepatic lipidosis is the most common form of liver dysfunction in cats. It can occur spontaneously (idiopathic), but most often it occurs as a consequence of anorexia caused by another underlying disease. Such diseases include inflammatory bowel disease, alimentary lymphoma, lymphocytic or neutrophilic cholangitis, pancreatitis, diabetes, chronic kidney disease, feline lower urinary tract disease, and stress. Overweight cats are predisposed.

Clinical signs

- Anorexia, weight loss.
- Jaundice.
- Dehydration.
- Vomiting.
- Signs of hepatic encephalopathy (hypersalivation, depression).
- Hepatomegaly.

Diagnosis

- Marked increase in ALP. Variable increases in ALT and total bilirubin.
- Serum biochemistry profile often reveals decreased liver function (low albumin, BUN, and cholesterol; high total bilirubin).
- Hepatomegaly on radiographs. Hyperechoic liver on ultrasound.
- Liver cytology: vacuolated hepatocytes.
- Liver biopsy may be needed.

> 50%–95% of cats with hepatic lipidosis have an underlying condition that resulted in anorexia.

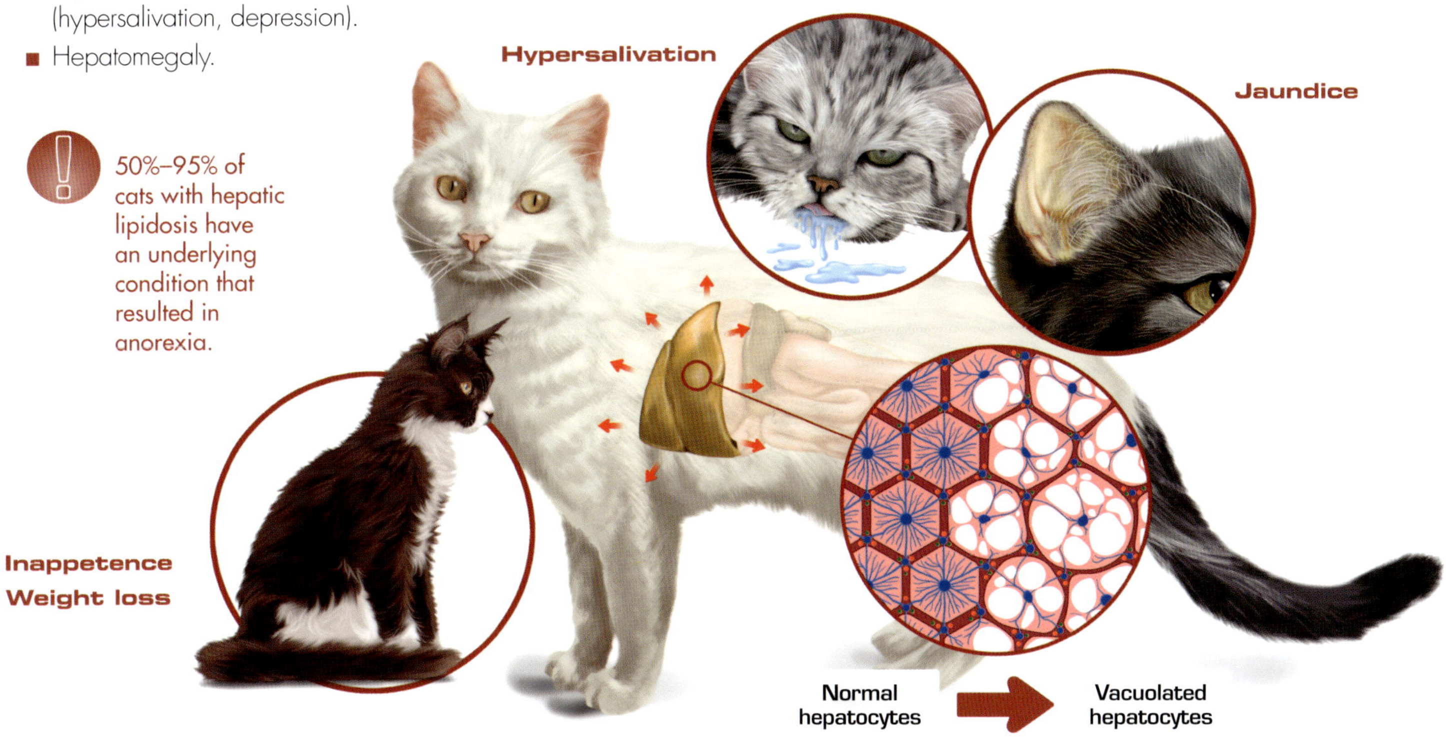

Treatment

- Aggressive enteral nutritional support and intravenous fluids.
- Treatment of any underlying conditions.
- Anti-nausea medications (e.g., ondansetron, maropitant) and appetite stimulants (e.g., mirtazapine, cyproheptadine).
- Treatment of hepatic encephalopathy (see Sheet 52).
- Treatment of bleeding tendencies with subcutaneous vitamin K_1 (rare risk of anaphylactic reaction).
- Hepatoprotectants (e.g., N-acetylcysteine, S-adenosylmethionine, ursodeoxycholic acid).
- Pain management in case of pancreatitis.

Prognosis

- Good if recognized early and treated appropriately.
- If not treated, hepatic lipidosis can be fatal.

> Aggressive nutritional support with a feeding tube is critical in the treatment of hepatic lipidosis.

DISEASES OF THE LIVER

64 Hepatic cancer

Primary liver tumors are rare in dogs and cats. Liver metastases are more common than primary liver tumors in the dog and tend to originate from cancer in the spleen, pancreas, or gastrointestinal tract. In cats, primary hepatobiliary tumors are more frequent, with biliary carcinomas being most common (see Sheet 51). Hepatocellular carcinomas are the most common primary tumor of the dog liver.

Clinical signs

- Patients may be asymptomatic or have nonspecific clinical signs.
- Anorexia, weight loss.
- Less frequent signs include vomiting, diarrhea, and increased thirst and urination.
- Acute weakness may be seen with bleeding masses.

Diagnosis

- Abdominal ultrasound may reveal a discrete tumor, multiple nodules, or diffuse enlargement of the liver.
- Liver biopsy for definitive diagnosis.

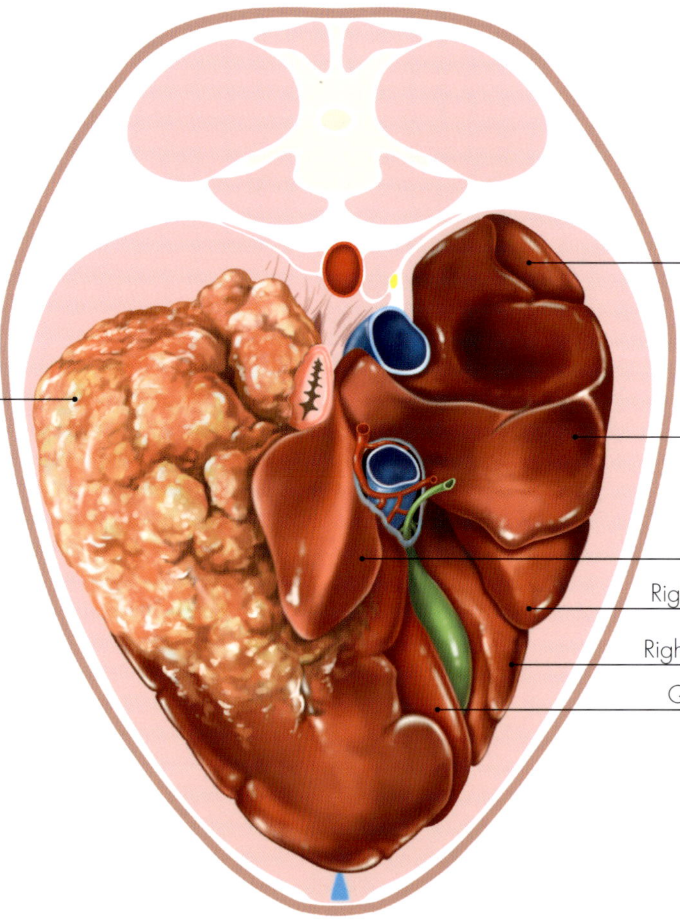

Treatment

- Surgery (liver lobectomy) for single, discrete hepatic masses (e.g., hepatocellular adenomas and carcinomas).
- Chemotherapy for diffuse cancers (e.g., lymphoma).

Prognosis

- Surgical removal of adenomas is curative.
- Surgical removal of isolated hepatocellular carcinomas may be curative; however, 37% of patients have metastasis at the time of the diagnosis.
- Diffuse hepatocellular carcinomas carry a poor prognosis: 100% of patients have metastasis at the time of diagnosis.
- Biliary carcinomas are aggressive, with metastasis in 80% of cases.
- Hepatosplenic lymphomas in dogs carry a poor prognosis.

65 Cholecystocentesis

Cholecystocentesis is aspiration of bile from the gallbladder.

Indications

- Evaluation of bile for evidence of hepatobiliary infection.

Contraindications

- Gallbladder mucocele.
- Extrahepatic bile duct obstruction.
- Coagulopathy.

Types

- **Ultrasound-guided:** using ultrasound guidance, a needle is inserted through the skin and into the gallbladder.
- **Laparoscopic:** using a small, specialized camera inserted into the abdominal cavity, the gallbladder is visualized and a needle is guided through the skin and into the gallbladder.
- **Surgical:** the gallbladder is held as a needle is carefully inserted into it under direct visualization.

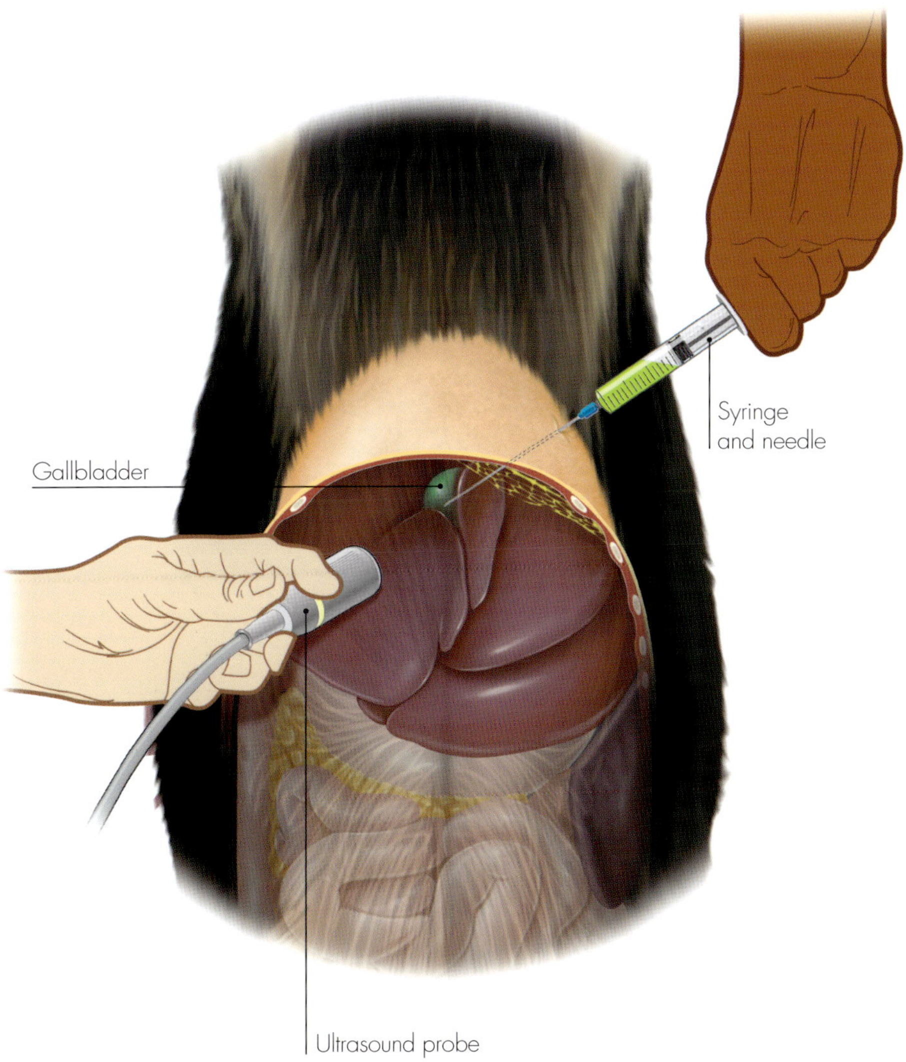

Procedure

- The patient is heavily sedated (ultrasound-guided cholecystocentesis) or placed under general anesthesia.
- A needle is inserted into the gallbladder and gentle suction is applied to the syringe.
- When possible, the entire gallbladder is emptied to lessen chances of bile leakage.
- Suction is released from the syringe and the needle is removed.

Evaluation of samples

- Cytological evaluation: identification of bacteria and abnormal cells.
- Bacterial culture and sensitivity.

Possible complications

- Bile peritonitis (leakage of bile into the abdomen).
- Rupture of the gallbladder.
- Vasovagal reaction (sudden and life-threatening decrease in heart and respiratory rates).

66 Laparoscopic liver biopsy

Laparoscopic liver biopsy is a minimally invasive procedure performed under anesthesia to collect samples for evaluation of various liver diseases. Laparoscopy offers advantages such as decreased pain, improved cosmesis, quicker recovery, and improved visualization and magnification.

Indications

- Investigate acute and chronic hepatopathies.

Contraindications

- Disease of the common bile duct or gallbladder that may necessitate a decompressive procedure.

Procedure

- Performed under general anesthesia.
- A camera is passed through a small incision in the skin just behind the umbilicus.
- The liver and gallbladder are evaluated.
- Another small incision is made in the skin on the left or right side to allow the insertion of instruments (e.g., probe, biopsy forceps).
- Four or five liver samples are taken for:
  - Histopathology.
  - Heavy metal (e.g., copper) quantification.
  - Culture.
- Bile is often collected percutaneously under laparoscopic guidance.

Possible complications

- Excessive bleeding.
- Pain.
- Splenic laceration.
- Gallbladder rupture.

Some complications (e.g., splenic laceration, excessive bleeding) may warrant conversion to an open surgical approach.

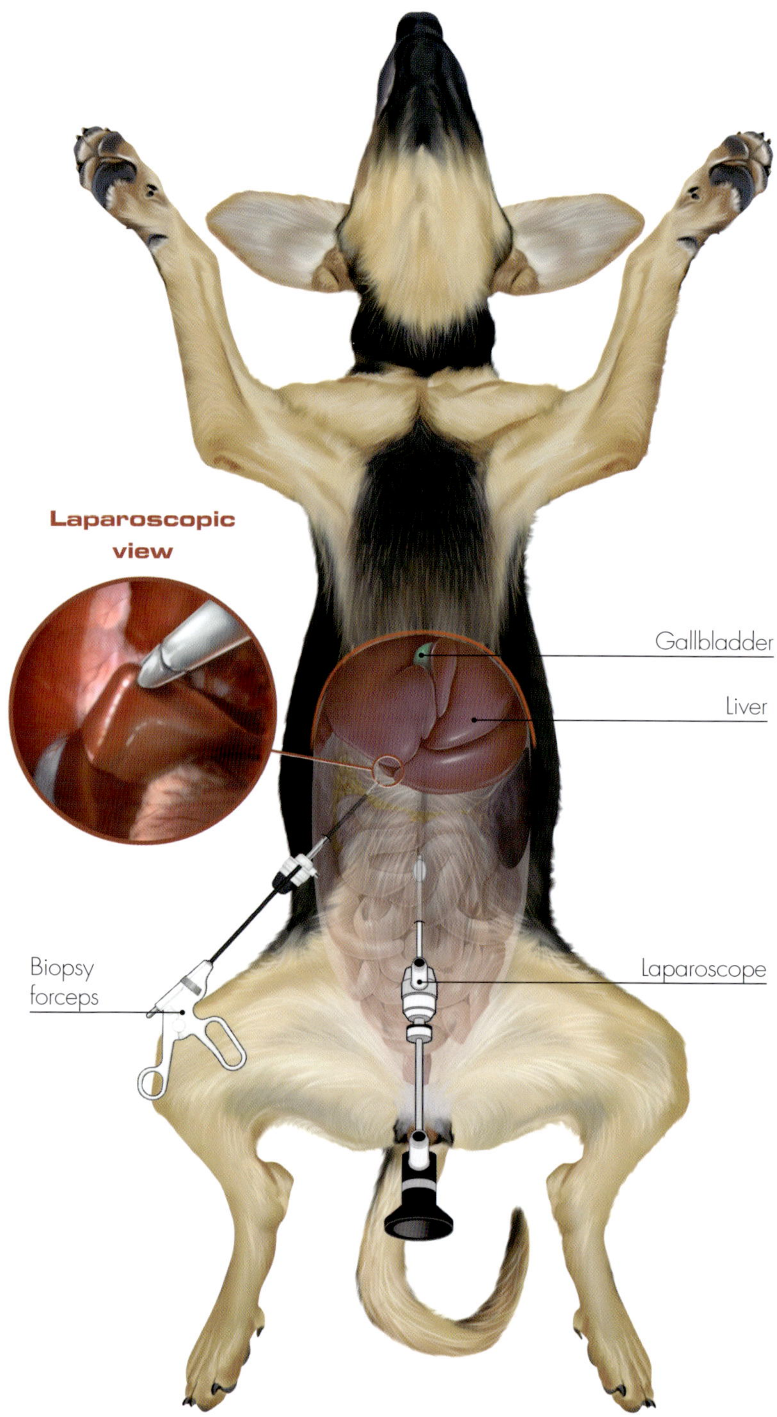

67 Anatomy of the pancreas

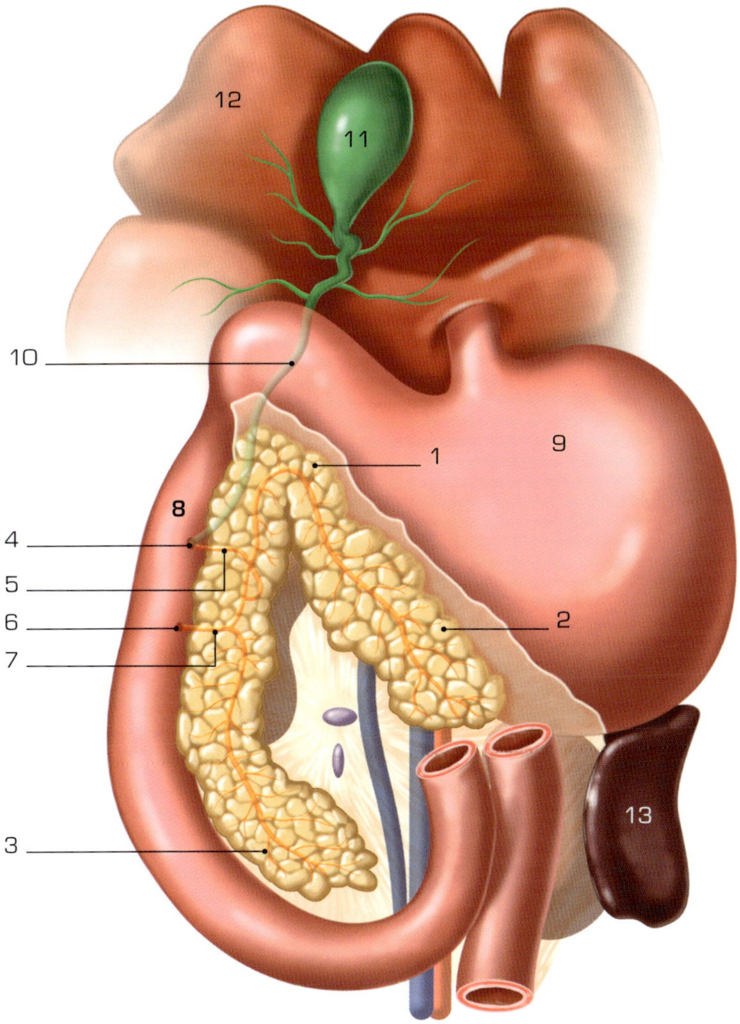

1. Body of the pancreas
2. Left lobe of the pancreas
3. Right lobe of the pancreas
4. Major duodenal papilla
5. Pancreatic duct
6. Minor duodenal papilla
7. Accessory pancreatic duct
8. Duodenum
9. Stomach
10. Common bile duct
11. Gallbladder
12. Liver
13. Spleen

Dogs have both pancreatic and accessory pancreatic ducts, with the latter predominating. Only 20% of cats have an accessory pancreatic duct.

Dog

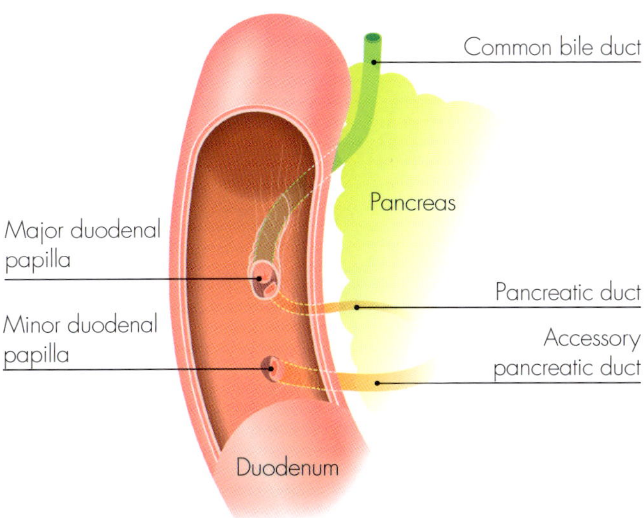

Cat

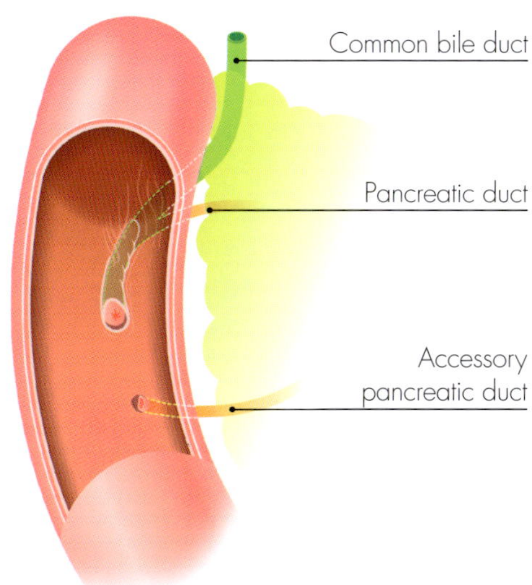

68 Physiology of the pancreas

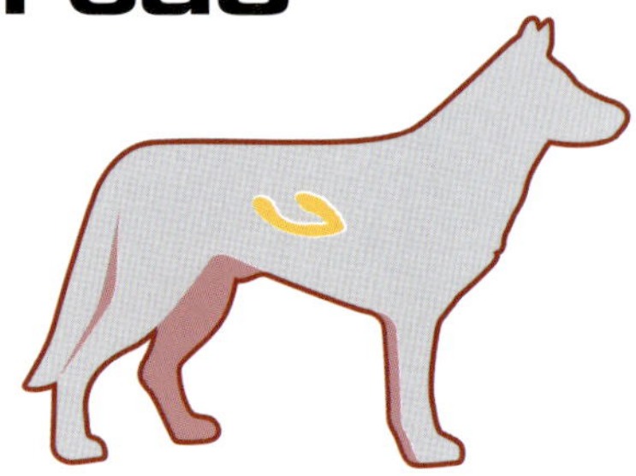

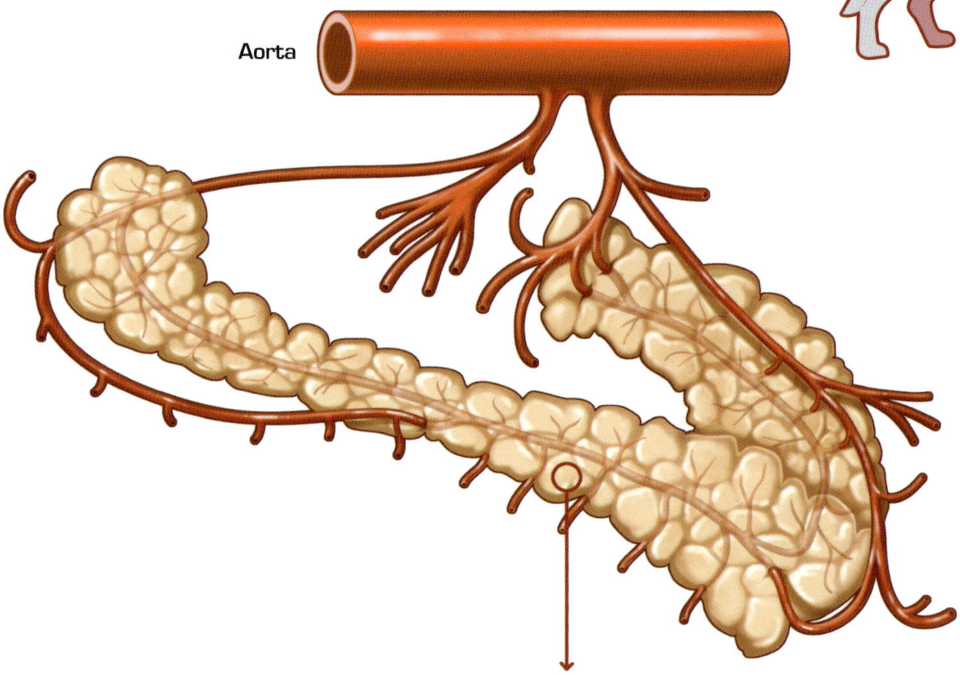

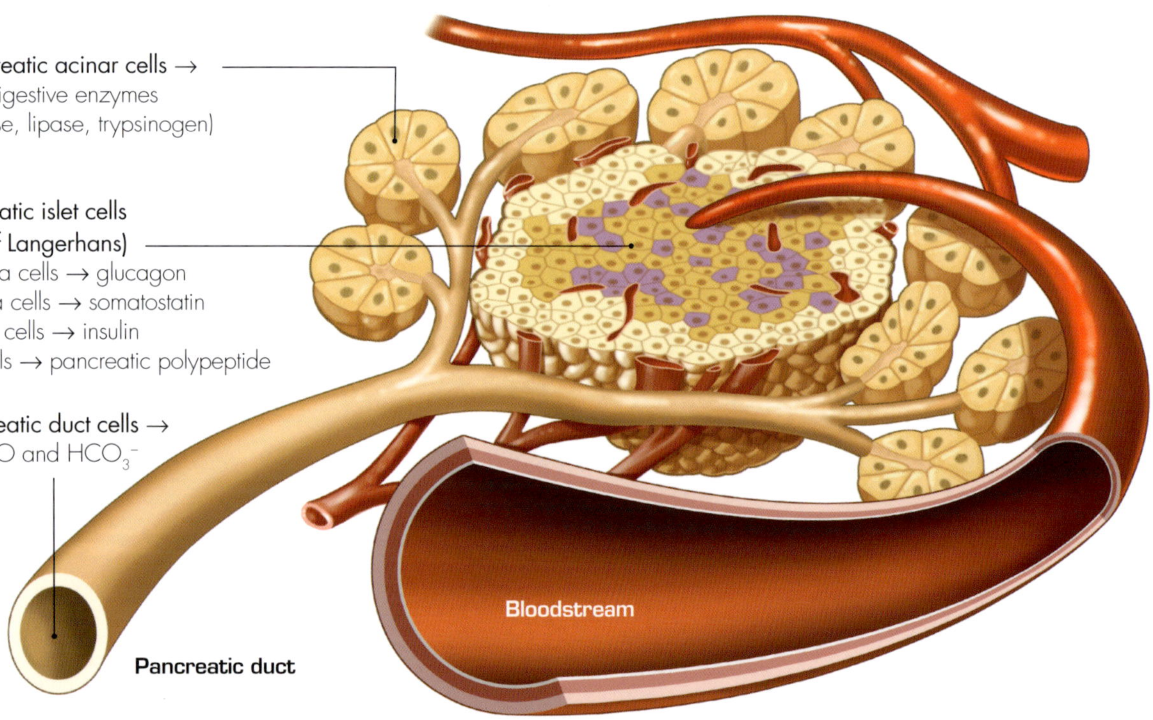

69 Exocrine pancreatic insufficiency (EPI)

In dogs, EPI most often occurs secondary to idiopathic atrophy (young dogs, average 1–4 years) or immune-mediated destruction (middle-aged to older animals) of pancreatic exocrine acinar cells. German Shepherd Dogs are overrepresented, but EPI can occur in any breed. Cats of any age can develop EPI, and it is thought to develop secondary to recurrent pancreatitis. Pets with EPI can develop intestinal dysbiosis.

Clinical signs

- Weight loss despite a normal to ravenous appetite.
- Small bowel diarrhea.
- Steatorrhea (fatty stools).
- Flatulence.
- Vomiting.

Diagnosis

- Abdominal ultrasound cannot diagnose EPI but is helpful in looking for pancreatic masses or changes consistent with pancreatitis in older dogs and cats.
- Documentation of a low trypsin-like immunoreactivity (TLI) after an 8–12 hour fast.
  - Dogs: <2.5 μg/dl.
  - Cats: <8.0 μg/dl.
- Evaluation of serum cobalamin and folate.

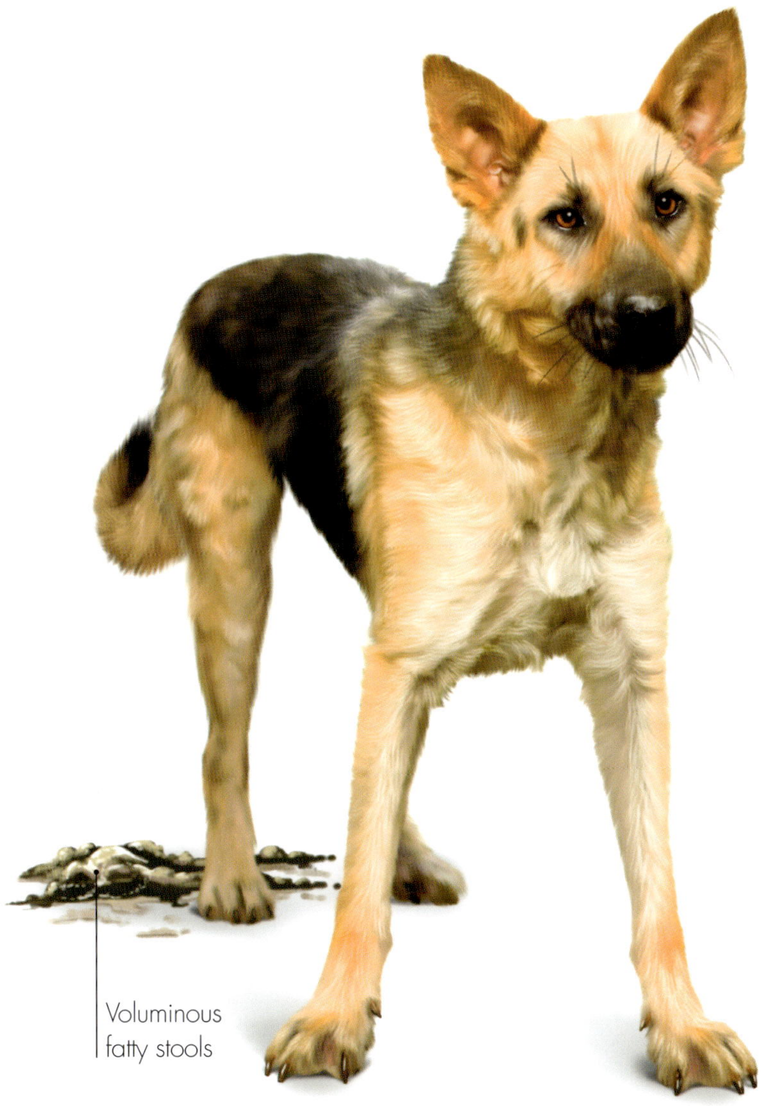

Low cobalamin is common in dogs and cats with EPI.

Treatment

- Oral administration of pancreatic enzymes (may be mixed with food).
- Supplementation of cobalamin when indicated.
- Treatment of dysbiosis with probiotics and/or tylosin may be necessary.

Treatment with pancreatic enzymes does not affect TLI, such that it can be evaluated even if the pet was already started on pancreatic enzymes.

Prognosis

- Good.
- Patients that have an incomplete response may need treatment for intestinal dysbiosis.

70 Acute pancreatitis

Acute inflammation of the pancreas, or pancreatitis, is common in dogs. It can occur in any age, breed, or sex, but Miniature Schnauzers and Yorkshire Terriers appear to be at an increased risk. In many cases, the cause of pancreatitis is unknown. However, some causes of pancreatitis in dogs include ingestion of high-fat food, dietary indiscretion (e.g., eating trash), hypertriglyceridemia, genetics/breed predisposition, obesity, severe blunt trauma, certain medications (e.g., potassium bromide, phenobarbital, azathioprine), underlying endocrine disease (e.g., diabetes mellitus, hyperadrenocorticism, hypothyroidism), and complications of anesthesia or abdominal surgery.

Clinical signs

- Vomiting.
- Anorexia.
- Abdominal pain.
- Diarrhea.
- Jaundice.

Diagnosis

- Abdominal ultrasound may reveal a hypoechoic pancreas with hyperechoic surrounding fat and tissue (68% sensitivity).
- Species-specific pancreatic lipase immunoreactivity (PLI).

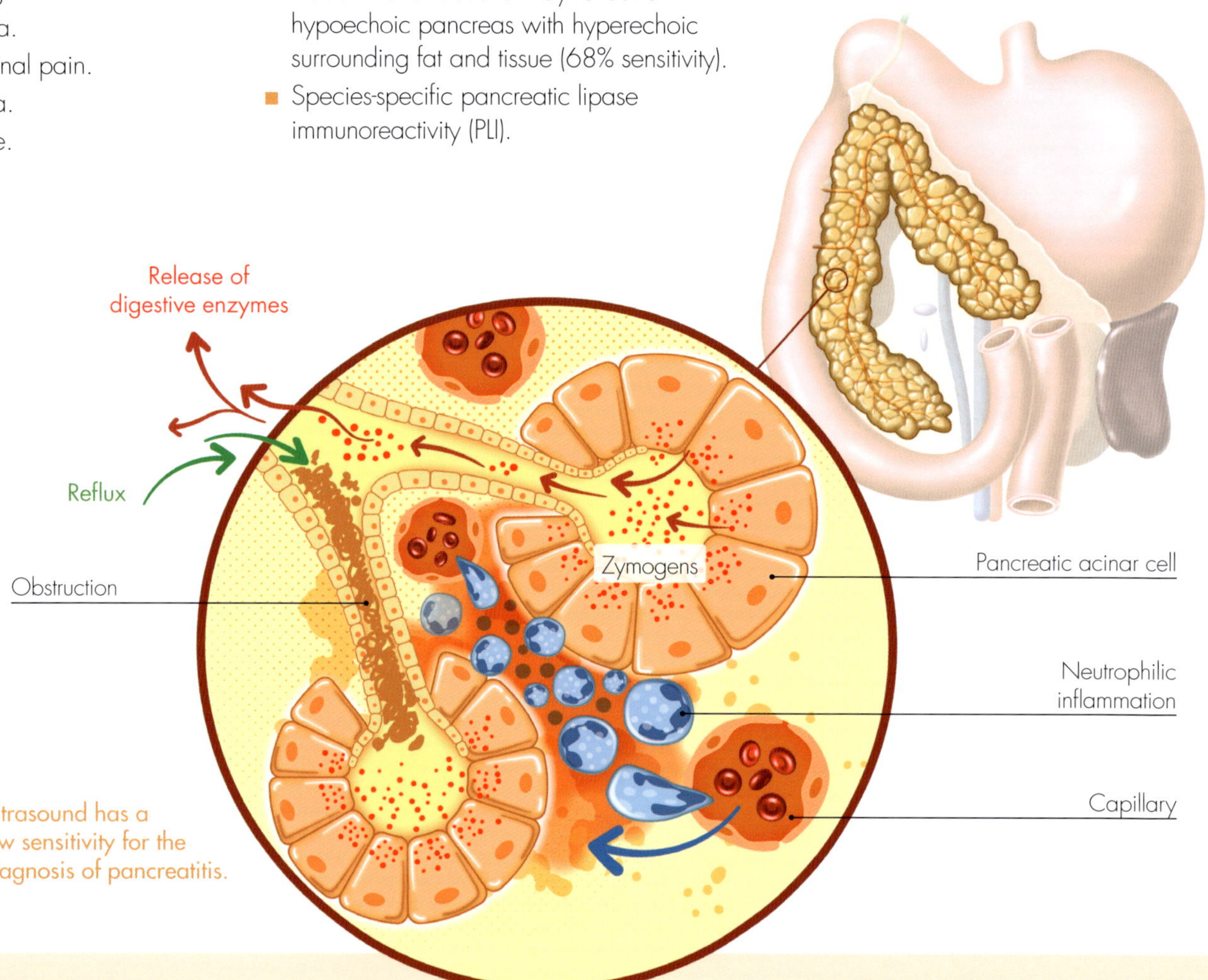

Ultrasound has a low sensitivity for the diagnosis of pancreatitis.

Treatment

- Supportive care with intravenous fluid therapy, pain management, anti-nausea medications, and early enteral nutritional support.
- A low-fat diet (<30 g fat/1000 kcal ME) is recommended for dogs with pancreatitis.
- Treatment of underlying diseases if possible.
- Surgery may be necessary for dogs with complications such as pancreatic abscesses, necrotic masses, or extrahepatic bile duct obstruction.

Prognosis

- Highly variable.
- Good in mild cases.
- Guarded for dogs with severe pancreatitis, pancreatic complications (e.g., pancreatic abscess), or concurrent diseases (e.g., diabetes mellitus).

71 Chronic pancreatitis

Chronic pancreatitis is defined as an inflammatory disease of the pancreas characterized by irreversible morphologic changes that cause loss of function and pain. Fibrosis (scar tissue) within the pancreas reduces the distensibility of this organ, resulting in duct blockage during secretion of digestive enzymes. As a result, recurrent bouts of acute pancreatitis occur, leading to further loss of functional pancreatic tissue. Once greater than 80% of functional pancreatic mass is lost, this loss of function may progress to exocrine pancreatic insufficiency or diabetes mellitus.

Clinical signs

- Intermittent, mild gastrointestinal signs (anorexia, vomiting, diarrhea, abdominal pain).
- Signs of acute pancreatitis may be present.

Diagnosis

- Exclusion of predisposing diseases (e.g., diabetes mellitus, intestinal disease).
- Ultrasound often reveals a hyperechoic and/or irregular pancreas that may have mass-like changes.
- Serum cobalamin, folate, and pancreatic lipase and trypsin-like immunoreactivity.
- Pancreatic biopsy for definitive diagnosis (rarely done).

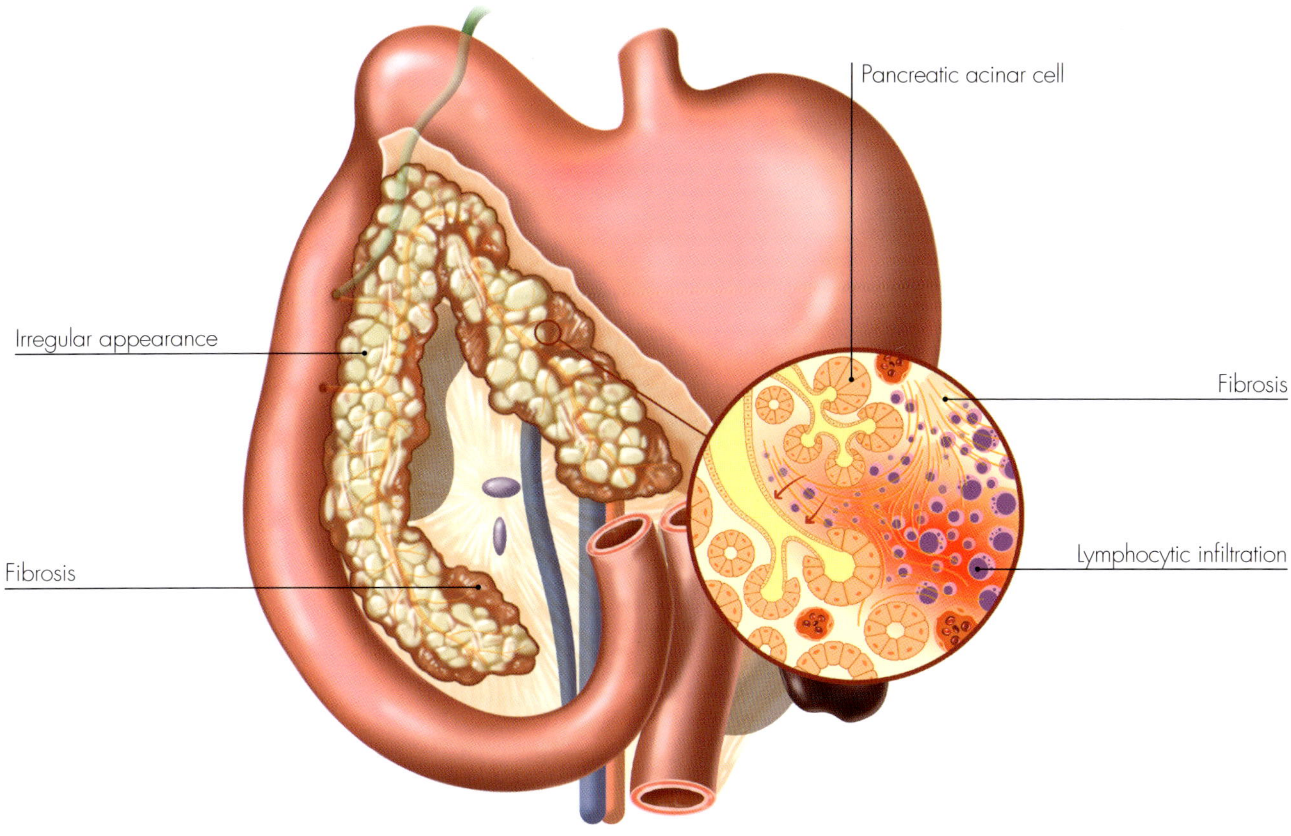

Treatment

- Management of recurrent bouts of acute pancreatitis (see Sheet 70).
- Pain management.
- Lifelong low-fat diet in dogs.
- Treatment of hyperlipidemia in dogs (e.g., low-fat diet, bezafibrate).
- Treatment of underlying inflammatory bowel disease in cats (e.g., hydrolyzed or novel protein diet, immunosuppressants).
- Monitoring for and addressing loss of pancreatic function.

Prognosis

- Highly variable.
- Good in pets with diet-responsive disease.
- Guarded in pets with frequent acute episodes or complicating diseases.

72 Pancreatic abscesses and pseudocysts

Pancreatic abscesses and pseudocysts are reported complications of acute and chronic pancreatitis. They occur infrequently in dogs and cats and are most often sterile. Pancreatic abscesses are a collection of pus, or white blood cells, whereas pancreatic pseudocysts contain a collection of enzyme-rich pancreatic fluid.

Clinical signs

- Small pseudocysts are clinically asymptomatic.
- Mild, intermittent gastrointestinal signs.
- Signs of acute pancreatitis (see Sheet 70).

Diagnosis

- Abdominal ultrasound: fluid-filled structure in association with the pancreas.
- Fine needle aspiration to collect fluid from within the abscess or pseudocyst for cytological evaluation and culture.
- Evaluation for acute or chronic pancreatitis (species-specific pancreatic lipase immunoreactivity).

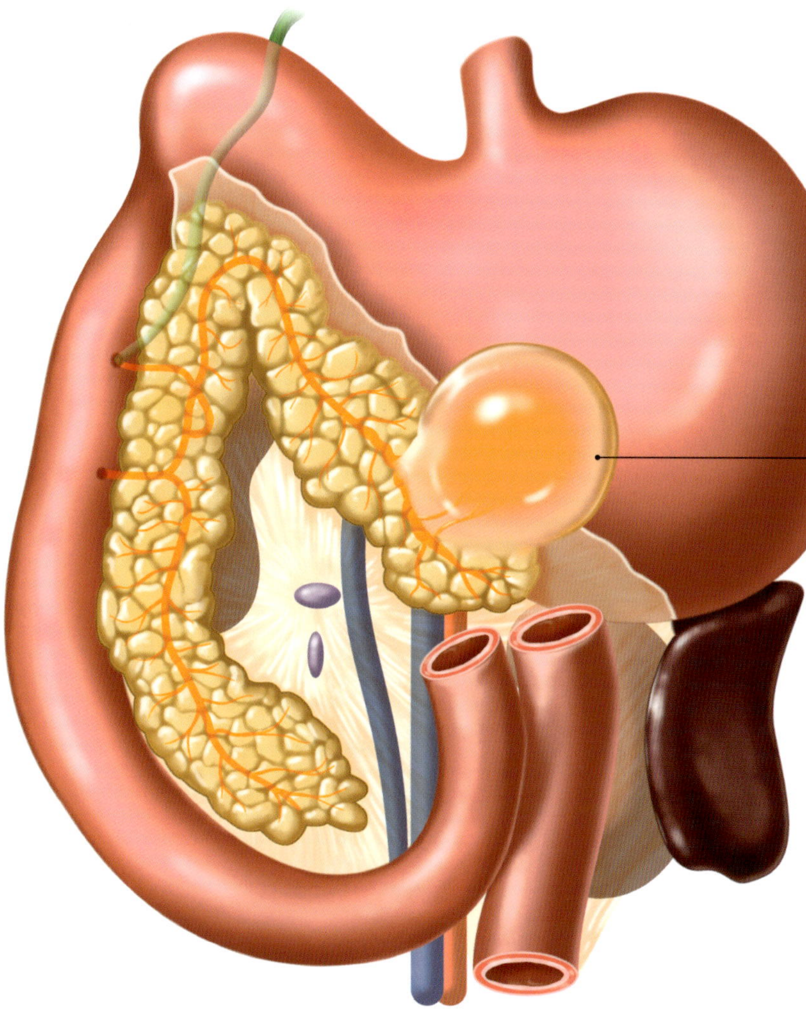

Treatment

- Medical management of pancreatitis (see Sheet 70).
- Sterile abscesses and pseudocysts can be drained using ultrasound guidance, but they often refill. Surgical intervention may be necessary for rapidly enlarging pseudocysts.
- Surgical drainage and aggressive antibiotic therapy for infected pancreatic abscesses and pseudocysts.

Prognosis

- Generally good.
- Fair to grave in pets that require surgical drainage for infected pancreatic abscesses.

73 Pancreatic cancer

Carcinomas are the most common pancreatic tumor in dogs and cats. They behave aggressively, with a high metastatic rate. Adenomas, which have only been reported in cats, are usually incidental and benign.

Clinical signs

- Anorexia.
- Weight loss.
- Vomiting.
- Abdominal effusion or mass effect.
- Jaundice if causing extrahepatic bile duct obstruction.
- Paraneoplastic alopecia in cats.

Diagnosis

- Abdominal ultrasound to visualize pancreatic masses.
- Fine needle aspiration of the pancreatic mass for cytology.
- Cytology of any free abdominal fluid.
- Pancreatic biopsy for definitive diagnosis.

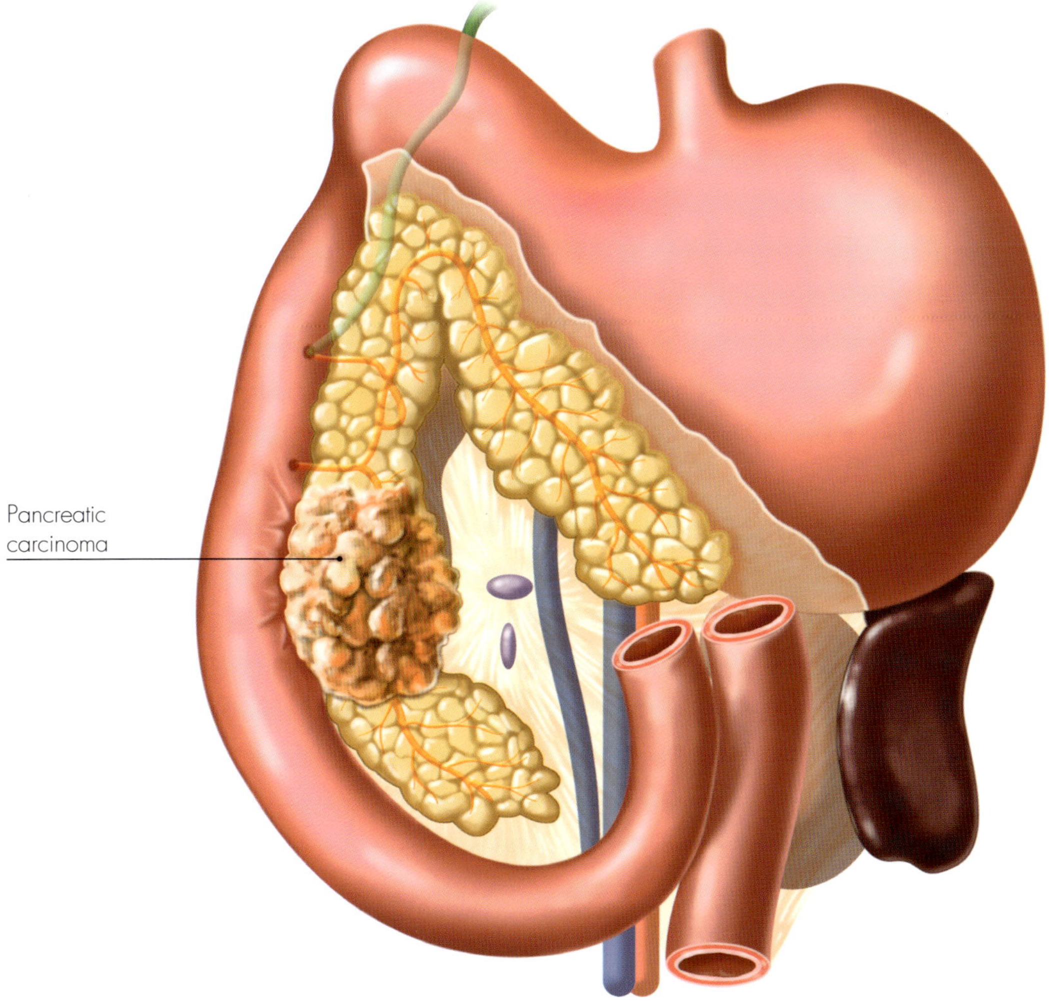

Treatment

- Surgical excision via partial pancreatomy for pancreatic carcinomas.
- Chemotherapy.

Prognosis

- Pancreatic carcinomas are highly aggressive and carry a poor prognosis; most pets are euthanized shortly after diagnosis due to metastasis and disease progression.